MAKE *Nutrition* FUN

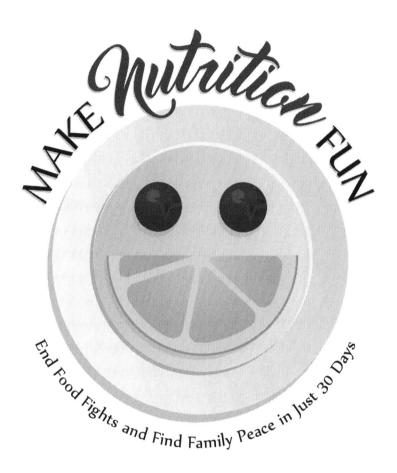

End Food Fights and Find Family Peace in Just 30 Days

D1377975

KATHRYN KEMP GUYLAY

Author photo by Christina Carlson.

Published by Healthy Solutions of Sun Valley, LLC

This book may be purchased in bulk, with special discounts, for educational, business, organizational, or promotional use. For information, please email: kg@MakeWellnessFun.com

Library of Congress Control Number: 2017950843

ISBN-13: 978-0-9965328-8-4

DEDICATION

To the tens of thousands of children and adults who have participated in Nurture programs over the past decade.

Thank you for reminding me, showing me, and practicing with me how to *make nutrition fun.*

About Nurture: Nurture is a nonprofit organization that provides nutrition education to children and families in a fun, hands-on way. Through partnerships and collaborations with food pantries, social services agencies, community organizations, and schools, our programs create long lasting behavior change for improved health and happiness. For more information about Nurture, please visit www.nurtureyourfamily.org.

SENDING YOU GRATITUDE

Thank you so much for buying this book. As an expression of my gratitude, I would like to offer you the cookbook of recipes from this book for FREE!

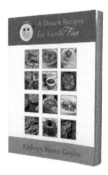

TO DOWNLOAD:

www.MakeNutritionFun.com/recipebook

You can also download a colorful 30-day calendar to commit to the Make Nutrition Fun challenge. The Make Nutrition Fun challenge includes 10 family fun activities and 15 recipes. Wow!

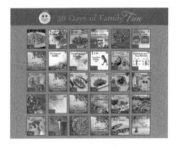

TO DOWNLOAD:

www.MakeNutritionFun.com/calendar

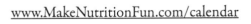

TABLE OF CONTENTS

Foreword

As a busy mom of three young girls (five years old and under), I am always on the lookout for fun and easy tips to help my family eat better.

After giggling my way through the first chapter of *Make Nutrition Fun: End Food Fights and Find Family Peace in Just 30 Days*, I couldn't put this book down. Kathryn offers up many excellent tips on how to raise healthy eaters without shame or extremes.

Furthermore, 30 days is the perfect amount of time to keep the family engaged. As a Registered Dietitian with decades of experience in family nutrition, I can attest that change needs to be specific and deliberate over a period of several weeks. Research shows that it takes about 30 days for neurological rewiring to support habit change.

Make Nutrition Fun is a month-long series of daily steps, organized by the alphabet. The fact that Kathryn gives us four days to catch our breath during this 30-day adventure (she has reflection and organization days for days 7, 14, 21, and 28) is a testament to her "progress over perfection" attitude. Her engaging stories and tips really do make nutrition fun. I love the colorful calendar that accompanies this book—the recipes and activities really support positive changes throughout the month and beyond.

I was introduced to Kathryn in 2007 when we both lived in Chicago. I was looking for friends that shared an interest in health and fitness and also to get involved in a community health initiative. I had heard about Kathryn and the nonprofit she founded, Nurture, and was intrigued by the concept of offering nutrition education disguised as hands-on cooking classes for at-risk and vulnerable populations. Given my background in community health at both the Project Healthy Schools research team at University of Michigan and the Poudre Valley Health Systems' Healthy Kids Club, I offered to help Kathryn and Nurture to develop the kids' nutrition programs.

When I first pulled up to Kathryn's house, I was happy to find a mom that raised her own chickens and grew a beautiful vegetable garden. Our friendship was sealed during our first walking meeting. Over the years, we continued our walk-and-talks, as the Nurture program and our friendship blossomed. Since inception, Nurture has served tens of thousands of people, providing interactive nutrition education, food equipment, and training to schools, community centers, and food banks.

My passion for healthy eating and career in nutrition stem from an early experience in life that taught me to tune-in to how foods make my body feel. When I look back at my childhood, my diet didn't exactly paint a picture of health. In fact, cookies, chips, soda, ice cream, and cake were my five food groups! Although I was a healthy weight, thanks to non-stop activity, the outside appearance was deceiving. I struggled with frequent stomachaches, anxiety, and IBS. When I was eight years old, a doctor suggested I keep a food journal to see if there were any obvious culprits. After one day of journaling, it was clear that the cake, cookies, and doughnuts were not helping. I continued to journal and noticed a huge improvement in my tummy troubles by limiting—but not eliminating—sweet treats. I learned that balance is key and that change should be gradual rather than abrupt.

In order to get the family on board, change needs to be **fun.** Kathryn does not disappoint in this department. Her activities are engaging, her recipes are delicious, and her advice is both kid and mamma-friendly.

Inside this book you'll find priceless nuggets of information and strategies that will transform your and your family's relationships with food. You'll also enjoy all the additional resources—recipes, activities, audio files, and more.

If you want to take your Make Nutrition Fun journey a

step further, join Kathryn and me at Make Nutrition Fun (www.MakeNutritionFun.com), where we provide even more recipes, resources, and online courses, customized to your needs.

In good health,

Juliette Britton, MS RD

Recipe Listing

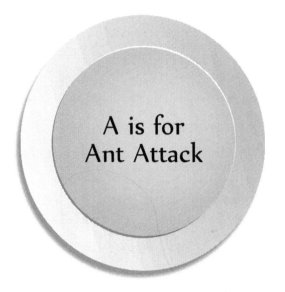

Day One

A is for Ant Attack

Around the time that my younger child, Alexander, was three, ants attacked my kitchen. Well, not exactly.

We were invited to a birthday party for my dear friend, Julia. We were in charge of bringing a cake and, given that Julia was one of the most accomplished cooks I knew, I felt pressured to find a recipe that would have a wow factor. My friend Chase had recently invited us over for dinner and, for dessert, had served a Bundt cake with a delicious chocolate glaze in a beautiful pattern dripping down the sides. Chase had five kids, so I knew she didn't mess around with complicated recipes.

"Just melt some dark chocolate and add a tiny bit of olive oil to give it a smooth texture," Chase said. "Then drip it down the cake in a pretty pattern. It is sure to impress!"

On the day of the party, 30 minutes before we had to leave, I was in the kitchen following Chase's instructions. I had the help and full attention of Alexander as we poured the dark chocolate over the cake.

"Great job, Alexander!" I said, as we finished the glaze. It was just starting to harden, and I did think that it would look beautiful.

"I am just going to go upstairs to take a quick shower before we go to the birthday party," I told Alexander. He nodded solemnly, pretending to go off to the playroom to busy himself.

About 15 minutes later, I came downstairs to find a boy with wide eyes and a huge ring of chocolate around his mouth.

"Mama. The ants. They came. And ate the cake!"

Very seriously, he led me to the kitchen, where the cake stood, yellow and pockmarked. There was not a morsel of chocolate to be found.

"Look, mama. See? The ants!"

I looked at my darling son, with his huge ring of chocolate around his mouth, and remembered the DO NOT EAT signs my stepmother used to hang on jars of chocolate chips. As a teenager, I had felt a lot of shame and guilt taking chocolate chips from those containers. I didn't want him to feel that same way.

"The ants did like that cake, didn't they?" I said with a smile. "Let's go wash your face, okay?"

I got on the phone with Julia and gave her the quick story, which elicited huge giggles.

"Okay, I'm good with the half-eaten cake ... Let's go with it." Julia was not only a superb cook, she was also a great sport.

We arrived at Julia's birthday with the cake, and all enjoyed a lovely meal. Our mealtime stories included the mystery of the ant attack on the cake. As the meal progressed, I noticed that Alexander was wobbling in his chair with half-closed eyes. I think he was stuffed full and hitting the sugar low at the same time. I refrained from chuckling, and no one scolded or judged. That day, Alexander learned his own, very personal and memorable lesson about how what you eat translates into how you feel. Now a teenager himself, Alexander must make his own decisions about what to eat, based on how the foods actually make him feel.

DAY 1 DOSE OF FUN

Avoid shame for a healthy long-term game

MORE MAGIC

Identify if you have any shame about food. Your feelings could stem from a childhood experience or might be something more current.

Now, go to that shameful feeling or moment and fully embrace it for what it's worth—an opportunity for you to make the best of a difficult situation. Forgive yourself and others for anything shameful that you might have previously associated with food. Remember that food is fuel, not bad or sinful.

Now, can you even laugh about that shameful feeling or experience?

Let go of shame and bring a little playfulness into your relationship with food. That is when you can really make nutrition fun.

If you'd like to learn more about how to avoid shame when talking about food with kids, I'd love to invite you to listen to an interview I hosted with Holistic Health Coach Kami Miller. Visit www.kathrynguylay.com/Kami to get a downloadable interview delivered right to your inbox.

Note: The moment that I fell deeply in love with my husband, Jeff, was when he first visited the home I lived in as a teenager. After being very gracious and socializing with my dad and stepmom, the two of us retreated alone to the kitchen. He saw the (same!?) jar of chocolate chips with the (same!?) DO NOT EAT sign, and he almost doubled over with laughter as he chuckled, "That's ridiculous". He walked directly over to the jar, opened it, reached in for a huge fistful, threw back his head, and dumped the entire handful into his mouth. I was hooked.

Recipe

. . . .

Ant Cake
(Bundt Cake with Chocolate Glaze)

POUND CAKE

Ingredients:

- 1 ½ cups butter, softened
- 1 8-ounce package cream cheese, softened
- 3 cups sugar
- 1 ½ teaspoon vanilla
- 3 cups flour (our adaptation was to divide between whole wheat and white flours)
- 6 eggs

Directions:

Spray and flour Bundt pan. Do not pre-heat oven. Blend butter and cream cheese until fluffy. Add sugar and vanilla. Alternate adding flour and eggs. Pour batter into pan. Place in a cold oven and heat it to 300 degrees. Bake for 1 hour and 35 minutes or until it cracks a bit on top. Cool.

CHOCOLATE GLAZE

Ingredients:

- 6 ounces high-quality chocolate chips
- 2 tablespoons mild tasting extra virgin olive oil

Directions:

Melt the chocolate the easiest way you can. We put it in a microwave-safe bowl and heat for 30 seconds at a time, stirring with a fork in between, until it is just melted. You can also melt the chocolate in a heatproof bowl set over a pan of simmering water. (The latter method was too high maintenance for me when my kids were small).

Once the chocolate is melted, stir in the olive oil until well blended and the glaze is smooth. While it is still liquid, pour the chocolate over the cooled Bundt cake in a pretty pattern, so that it drips down the side. Allow the chocolate to set at room temperature for about 15 minutes, then refrigerate.

Caution: This recipe may attract ants.

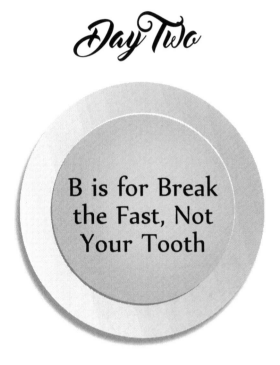

Day Two

B is for Break the Fast, Not Your Tooth

"Breakfast. Gotta start your day with breakfast!" my dad, Dr. Robert Kemp, cheerfully reminded us as he woke my sister and me in our hotel room.

As a biochemist, my dad ("Dr. Bob") frequently spoke at conferences around the world. My sister and I were always thrilled when he allowed us to tag along, mostly because we loved to lounge at the hotel pool. When we were teenagers, he had a conference in Puerto Rico during one of many long and frigid Chicago winters, so we begged him to let us come. He relented on the condition that we would not sleep until noon, as usual, but instead enjoy the fresh air and maybe even the historical sites. And, of course, we also had to listen to his biochemist views at mealtime.

"Protein makes up the building blocks of your body," he pontificated as we made our way down the hall to breakfast. "Breakfast is the meal of champions," he continued.

So we made sure to get all of our macronutrients and as many micronutrients as we could at the breakfast bar. My dad was a sucker for Canadian bacon, which they offered in stacks at the hotel, so he was definitely going to get his protein.

As we sat down to eat, my sister asked my dad, "How many people are you speaking to today?"

"About a thousand," my dad answered. "So I'd better make sure that I don't have anything stuck in my teeth before I start." He dabbed his napkin against his professor-like face and looked at us in a very serious, ivory-tower way. Then, as he took a bite of his beloved Canadian bacon, there was a disturbing *CRACK* noise. His eyes grew wide, and he panicked as he looked around for his napkin. He stooped below the table and, as inconspicuously as possible, spit something into his napkin. When he sat upright again, he looked straight at my sister and me.

Gasp!

Having something stuck in his teeth was the *least* of my dad's worries. At the front of his smile sat an enormous black hole. He had just chipped off a huge chunk of his front tooth.

"Cool, Dad! You look just like Wayne Gretzky!" I said admiringly.

My dad looked at Suzanne, who had burst into an uncontrolled laugh.

"No, you look like Billy Bob!" Suzanne managed to say through her tears of laughter.

My dad was getting flustered. His talk was in 15 minutes. There was simply nothing he could do. He would have to make his keynote presentation as Dr. Billy Bob.

BUILD YOUR DAILY FOUNDATION WITH BREAKFAST

Now that you know about my biochemist Dad and his love for both protein and breakfast, let's dive into the concept of breakfast even further.

Breakfast literally means *break the fast*. To fast is to go without food for more than eight hours. Your body does this every night, assuming you don't raid the fridge at midnight, so it is important to fuel up in the morning before you set off on your busy day.

Without breakfast, you might start to feel sluggish or even get the shakes.

Breakfast can help you focus on your work and be more successful, whether that means better performance at school, increased productivity at work, or more positivity as a family and community member.

Here are some top reasons to eat breakfast:

- Breakfast gives your body energy and much-needed nutrients after the fast. Kids and adults who eat breakfast perform better in sports. The theory is that breakfast-skippers might not be getting the vitamins, minerals, and other nutrients they need.

- Breakfast starts up your metabolism in the morning, helping you to maintain a healthy weight. Getting into a meal routine helps to keep your appetite under control. Breakfast eaters are less likely to overeat at other meals or snacks.

- Meals in the morning can help to put you in a happier mood!

Breakfast should be made up of the following key components, listed here in order of importance:

1. Protein source. Dr. Billy Bob's advice was accurate. Protein provides the building blocks for our bodies. Without it, we can't sustain our strength. Always remember your protein.

2. Fruit or vegetable. We need to get at least five servings of fruits and vegetables every day, so why not start in the morning? Fruits and vegetables provide so many great nutrients—and are so delicious—it's important not to miss out.

3. Healthy fat. Add healthy oils, like olive oil, nuts, or avocado to your breakfast. Fats take a while to digest, so they keep you full longer. Fats have all kinds of good things in them like omega-3 fatty acids, the helpful kind that build a healthy brain. A simple trick to getting those omega-3s is to sprinkle ground flax seeds on anything you prepare. This addition is a nice way to change it up if you don't feel like adding olive oil, nut butter, or large seeds to your meal. (Note: Store ground flax seeds in the freezer, as they are particularly sensitive to becoming rancid.)

4. Whole grains. Note the word "whole." The advice to eat whole grains does not mean a white bagel or toast before you run out the door. If that's all you eat, you are likely to be out of energy and really hungry in an hour or two. Whole grains include all parts of the grain and are minimally processed, so your body will take its time converting them to energy. The USDA nutrition guidelines (MyPlate) tell us that half our grains should be whole, but I think the more the better. Whole grains include oatmeal, barley, quinoa, millet, brown rice, bulgur wheat, and many others.

DAY 2 DOSE OF FUN

Know the right way to structure the first meal of your day

MORE MAGIC

Don't like being a short order cook? Don't do it anymore! Instead, create a "breakfast bar" in the morning with the four ingredients outlined above. For example, just make one pot of steel cut oats (whole grains). Set out options for your family members from which they can choose. Try peanut butter, Greek yogurt, or whole nuts (which happen to cover both protein and healthy fats). Set out banana slices, apples, or raisins (or any fruit or vegetable). Feeling extra fun in the morning? Offer cinnamon or other favorite spices for your family members to add. Then let the fun set in as your family members invent their very own customized breakfast that they will actually eat and enjoy. In my house, the end result of my breakfast bar looks completely different from person to person. Apples, peanut butter, and oats for my son. Yogurt, berries, and oats for my daughter. Oats, nuts, milk, and raisins for my husband. It seems like several different menu options, but I only made one thing (oats). For me, making nutrition fun means no complaints, returns, re-work, or wasted food.

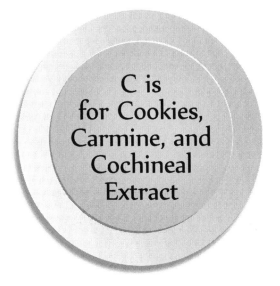

Day Three

C is for Cookies, Carmine, and Cochineal Extract

"Come on. Time to leave!" Jeff said as he finished packing up the car. We were planning a trip to the Grand Canyon, and we had many hours of driving ahead of us, including inevitable stops for snacks at gas stations.

I was ready with my car games.

"Okay, kids! Our first game is Food Ingredient Scavenger Hunt. You'll see the list of items on the first sheet in the activity packet I just handed you."

"There are *bugs* in our food?" my older child Elena asked. She is a fast reader.

"Yes! You are going to be looking for the word 'carmine' at our first gas stop. First one to find it gets five points!"

"Gross, Mom! The sheet says that carmine is made of cochineal extract from the female Dactylopius coccus *costa*." Her voice began to rise. "They are harvested mainly in Peru and the Canary Islands. The girl bugs eat pink cactus pads, and the color gathers in their bodies and eggs. Once harvested, dried, and ground, these bugs make their way into things like yogurt, frozen fruit bars, and fruit juice."

Alexander wanted to one-up his sister. "So what? A little bug juice never hurt anyone."

"Alexander! It says that carmine can cause allergic reactions in some people."

We got to our first gas station. To the dismay of all the customers, and certainly the guy working behind the counter, my kids ran in the door yelling, "Dead bugs! We're on the lookout for dead bugs!"

Elena was the winner of this round. She emerged from the gas station with a plastic wrapped cookie—Grandma's brand—in her hands. She was very proud of her find. She held onto that cookie for dear life throughout the entire round trip as it crumbled inside of the packaging. She was excited to show the bug cookie to her friends and teacher when she returned home.

"I can't believe Grandma put dead bugs in her cookies," Jeff said as we drove past that same gas station on the way back from the Grand Canyon.

"Yeah, Mom. We'll stick with your homemade ones from now on," my kids said to me as I smiled stealthily in the front seat.

DAY 3 DOSE OF FUN

Have a game of try-and-find-its,
but beware of gas station riots

MORE MAGIC

Can you come up with a scavenger hunt game that makes food education, shopping, cooking or even traveling fun? The more we can be playful in our education, the more the lessons will sink in.

It is important to recognize that allergens in food are something to consider as a factor in your child's behavior. People have asked me during talks I've given on nutrition, "What's the problem with the bug additives?" The answer is nothing, unless you or your family members are allergic to it. I have heard about a child having an anaphylactic reaction (when the airways are cut off) in her car seat after eating a food with the carmine additive. Allergies, both acute and chronic (like food intolerances), are things to be aware of. If you'd like to learn more about allergies and food sensitivities, I'd love to invite you to listen to a few interviews I've conducted with parents and experts on this topic. Visit the links below to get downloadable interviews delivered right to your inbox.

My interview with Amy Hager, Registered Dietitian, Nutritionist, Certified Diabetes Educator, and Certified Wellness Coach, is available at www.kathrynguylay.com/Amy.

With Ginger Hudock, holistic nutrition consultant, we talked about food sensitivities and much more: www.kathrynguylay.com/Ginger.

My interview with parent Trisha Hughes (creator of the website Eat Your Beets) is available at www.kathrynguylay.com/Trisha. Trisha helped her highly allergic baby heal from severe allergies by applying the GAPS diet.

Recipe

• •

The Famous Guylay Family Chocolate Chip Cookies

Ingredients:

- 4 sticks of butter, softened
- 1 ½ cups of white sugar
- 1 ½ cups of brown sugar
- 3 teaspoons of high quality vanilla extract
- ½ teaspoon salt
- 1 ½ teaspoons baking soda
- 4 eggs
- 1 cup quick (rolled) oats (you can process them in the Cuisinart if you like; sometimes we do and sometimes we don't)
- 1 ½ cups whole wheat flour
- 2 ½ cups whole wheat white flour
- 2 bags (around 11 ounces each) of high quality chocolate chips

Directions:

Preheat the oven to 350 degrees. Mix everything together to make the dough; add the chips last.

Then make into cookies on cookie sheets. If you are being expeditious, which we often are, just put dough into two large rectangular Pyrex dishes sprayed with olive oil spray. This recipe is for a double batch. Why make a single one? We always freeze the cookies anyway.

Cook at 350 degrees for anywhere between six to ten minutes—it depends on if you've made cookies, which are thinner (cook for six minutes), or if you've made "bars" that you'll cut from the Pyrex dishes (cook for ten minutes). In either case, don't let the cookies brown while they are in the oven. The trick is to watch them until they are just cooked enough and then get them out of the oven quickly! The cookies might look under-baked when you take them out, but they continue to cook for a bit after they are out of the oven. After they cool, we put them in the fridge to "gel" overnight if we make them in the Pyrex dishes, so we can cut them out without too much mess. Believe me, not over-baking the cookies is the secret to our family's cookie recipe success.

Day Four

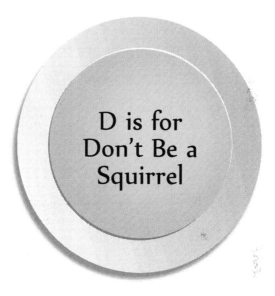

D is for Don't Be a Squirrel

"**D**addy! Look how cute it is!" said Elena, our family's animal lover. She was pointing at a grey squirrel that had run down a tree and was crossing the road. We were taking Elena to the park in a Baby Jogger stroller when she was just a toddler.

"Mommy, he's crossing the street! And there is a car!" said Elena with concern. Oh, no. The squirrel did that thing where it makes a choice and runs one way, then changes its mind and runs in the opposite direction, then back again. As it continued to second-guess itself, the car got closer and closer and closer.

Splat!

We turned our eyes away in horror. "WAAHHHHHHHH-HH!!" screamed Elena.

We pushed the stroller away from the scene of the crime as fast as we could. I knew we had a terrible day in front of us. Elena was heartbroken to see harm come even to the tiniest of ants. We knew the squirrel episode could be scarring for life.

"Stupid squirrel," said Jeff under his breath. "If only he could have just made up its mind."

THE SQUIRREL EFFECT DOES NOT MAKE NUTRITION FUN

It can be embarrassing to be in the field of nutrition in this day and age. We are a nation of squirrels ourselves, changing our minds over and over again about what is the right way to go. Low calorie? Higher calorie? Low fat? High fat? Low carb? High carb? Meat eating? Vegetarian? The contrasting list goes on and on. Nutritionists have given so much conflicting advice that we have confused the population and put them at as much risk as a clan of confused squirrels trying to cross a multi-lane highway. I am afraid that if we don't commit and engage with a solution, we will all go *splat* as well!

COMMITMENT CAN SAVE THE DAY

My antidote to the squirrel effect is to make a commitment. Choose one side of the road or the other, but base your decision on your own individual "gut check" and stick with it.

I started to really have fun with nutrition when I came up with my own personal system that made me feel good. My system is based mostly on the primal and Mediterranean eating principles; combined with a curiosity arising from *The Omnivore's Dilemma* (by Michael Pollan) about the food chain; polished with a desire to grow at least a portion of our family's food, from *Animal, Vegetable, Miracle* (by Barbara Kingsolver). My system is also holistic in the sense that wellness isn't just about food; it's also about movement, relationships, and even spirituality.

C   Connect to something greater than yourself.

O   Other people have a right to their own opinions.

M   Manage stress.

M   Move every day.

I   In Mother Earth, I trust.

T   Techniques for cooking should be simple.

M   Meals should be about friends and family.

E   Energy in, energy out.

N   Never say never.

T   Too much of a good thing can be harmful.

Here are some details about these ten components that make up my *commitment* to making nutrition fun.

1. Connect to something greater than yourself. It is no fun to feel alone. I don't think we are. If you are not religious, know that you can at least connect with Mother Nature. Try not to get too distracted by a myopic view of the world. Stop and remember that we are part of a vast, amazing universe.

2. Other people have a right to their own opinions. I have learned to avoid judging when it comes to food. I try really hard not to use the word "bad" when talking about food or nutrition. Arthur Agatston, author of *The South Beach Diet*, introduced me to the concept of good fats and good carbs, like olive oil, fruits and veggies, and whole grains. I love talking about food as good. It can be fun to rank a food in terms of how good it is. Agatston was the first to teach me about the glycemic index (GI), a measurement of a carb's effect on blood sugar. The GI scale goes from 0 to 100; the closer to zero, the less impact the food has on your blood sugar. Good carbs are lower on the glycemic index. They are digested slowly, so you feel fuller longer, and your blood sugar and appetite

don't go out of whack. Some carbs, like mashed potatoes, give you a blood sugar rush followed by a crash. Foods with a GI under 55 are considered low, between 56 and 69 intermediate, and those 70 and above are considered high. Understanding the GI scale is a great way to help you choose foods that will keep your energy steady throughout the day and avoid food-induced crashes.

If you want to evaluate your own food on the GI scale, I encourage it, but keep your findings to yourself. You might know that a plate of French fries can wreak havoc on your blood sugar, appetite, and energy level; but don't offer the information unless someone asks you. A friend scarfing down a side of fries might rather not know.

3. Manage stress. Nutrition is directly linked to 80 percent of morbidity factors, but stress is likely linked to 100 percent. The only two morbidity factors in the top 10 that I don't consider to be related to nutrition are accidents and suicide, which can easily be linked to stress. I encourage you to do what you need to manage stress in your life. The importance of stress management is a primary reason why I include mindfulness (see Day 15 about Mindful Eating) in this practice.

4. Move every day. My nickname in college was the Energizer Bunny, and I was known to buzz around campus nonstop. I also was a runner, especially once I began to recognize the positive effect running has on my mood.

Another huge factor that encouraged my running habit was my dog, Mackenzie, who pretty much forced me to run with him every day or he would destroy my tiny apartment. Need an incentive to run every day? Get a herding dog! Mackenzie kept me active throughout college, graduate school, work, and even in my early baby days.

I can't emphasize enough the importance of finding some way to get moving every single day. Exercise releases endorphins, the happy chemicals, in your brain. Keep trying methods of exercise until you find something that you absolutely love—dance, yoga, martial arts, hiking, walking, zumba, playing in the snow, biking, you name it! Talk to your doctor about starting an exercise program if you don't have one in place. Start with 15 minutes a day and work up to 60, if you can. An hour a day is the amount of physical activity recommended for kids, so go ahead and act like a kid.

5. In Mother Earth I trust. Please emphasize real food in your diet. Veggies should be your best friends. I also love nuts, seeds, and healthy oils, such as olive oil. I don't completely ban grains but stick to my favorites, which include quinoa and steel-cut oats. Strive to get protein with every meal in the form of eggs, dairy products, poultry, and fish, or plant- based sources, such as beans, seeds, nuts, and legumes. I'll eat red meat only on occasion.

If you're able, grow your own greens and herbs or buy local when available. There is nothing more satisfying than going out to your garden before dinner and cutting greens for a fresh salad. Grow or buy dark leafy greens (like chard, kale, or even the more adventurous tatsoi and mustard greens). Dark-green leafy vegetables are loaded with nutrients: folate, magnesium, trace minerals, vitamins A and K, and the kind of fiber that satisfies. If you are not used to eating dark greens, start with a mild green, such as romaine, and experiment from there.

In the Mediterranean plan, vegetables are tossed into almost everything, including soups, stews, sauces, salads, pasta, and pizza. They are often grilled and then drizzled with extra-virgin olive oil.

Support your local farmers and know from where your eggs, meat, and fish come. Take a trip to a farm with your kids and allow your experience to transform how much value you place on food. U.S. citizens spend much less on food as a percentage of income than most other countries. We have room to grow in this area.

6. Techniques for cooking should be simple. Simple cooking methods ensure that we eat home-cooked meals. Our family has home-cooked meals six nights a week, with one night at a restaurant (with a shared entrée, of course). I don't think that simple has to be boring. I'll talk more about how Rice Cookers (Day 20) and Slow Cookers (Day 22) can allow you to save tons of time and money on your make nutrition fun journey.

7. Meals should be about friends and family. Studies show that kids that eat dinner more often with their families get into less

trouble in their teen years. Try to sit down for a family dinner at least several times a week. Express gratitude for your food and eat slowly with pleasure and respect. Enjoy the company, too.

8. Energy in, energy out. I will save the details for our next chapter (Day 5), and I hope you'll enjoy the story about tug of war that reminds us to keep everything in balance.

9. Never say never. Guess how I start each and every day? With a small bowl of chocolate chips! No deprivation, and this special snack gives me motivation to get out of bed. I don't drink coffee, so a small amount of chocolate is my morning pick-me-up, even before I make breakfast. In the evenings, I don't hesitate to unwind with a delicious glass of wine, toasting with Jeff as we count our blessings. I never pass up an opportunity to taste a dessert, even if I might stick to only three bites. A happy hour, dinner, or dessert toast can be yet another chance to express gratitude in your day.

10. Too much of a good thing can be harmful. I'll get into more details on Day 23, but know that our bodies are hardwired to have a preference for sweet tastes. This kept our ancestors alive when they searched out berries and fruits at the end of a long winter; but in today's world of food abundance, the sweet tooth is something we need to be aware of and actively manage.

DAY 4 DOSE OF FUN

> *Make up your mind and be bold;*
> *don't go SPLAT in the middle of the road*

MORE MAGIC

What might your own commitment plan look like to make nutrition fun? My "commitment" is a long one, so maybe yours will be shorter and more simple. Be playful and creative and own your own plan. Allow enough flexibility in your plan that you can stick to it in the long term.

Sharkie Zartman, author of five books about getting active and healthy living, has a wonderful philosophy that has kept her looking young and feeling vibrant into her sixties. I'd like to invite you to listen to an interview I had with Sharkie that will give you actionable tips that perhaps you'll incorporate into your own commitment plan. Visit www.kathrynguylay.com/Sharkie to get a downloadable interview delivered right to your inbox.

Day Five

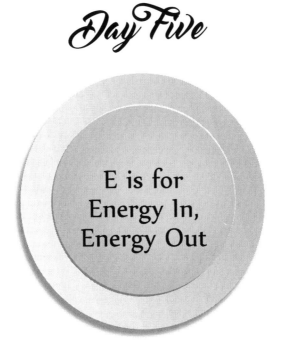

E is for
Energy In,
Energy Out

"Everyone gather around! Who likes to play tug-of-war?"

The group of kids who were previously avoiding me came over with fresh excitement and anticipation showing in their faces.

"Awesome. I'm so relieved," one of the kids said to me. "Our camp counselor said that it was time for some stupid nutrition and health lesson. We get to do this instead?"

"Yes!" I said with a smile, knowing that we were going to do both.

Separately, I made a mental note to track down the counselor later. If they wanted me to come and teach nutrition education to the camp kids, they were going to have to avoid the description "nutrition education".

"Let's get organized. Everyone is going to be assigned to either Team Food or Team Activity."

"Great! I'll be Team Food captain," a tall girl volunteered.

"Perfect. Now assign everyone on your team to be a specific food." I heard people shout out things like sandwich, fruit plate, granola bar, trail mix, and so on.

"I want to be Team Activity captain!" said a strong-looking boy.

"Sounds great. You assign everyone on your team to a specific activity." I heard him working with his teammates to assign activities such as soccer, swimming, walking the dog, gymnastics, and more.

I handed each of my team captains an end of the tug-of- war rope.

"Okay, you can add two foods to your side." Turning to the other captain, I said, "You can add two activities." The tug-of- war commenced.

We kept adding foods and activities with equal balance until we had about 15 kids on each side, pulling and pulling. The rope went back and forth a bit, but it was pretty steady. Then, it was time to make a statement.

"Okay, you activities," I said, pointing to about half the kids on one side, "you are now foods!" They ran over to the other side of the rope.

With an unequal distribution of power, the food side took over with such force that they all flew backwards into a mud puddle. I thought the kids would be mad at me for getting them covered in dirt, but I have never seen such fun and laughter, as these kids were thrilled to get dirty.

"I guess we overate," said the group in the mud puddle, laughing.

It was time to drive the lesson home. "Tell me what you think this game tells you about nutrition," I said.

One of the captains said, "To be healthy, we must balance the energy we put in our bodies—food—with what we burn through activities."

The other team captain added, "I guess weight gain happens when we put more food in than we need for activity. To build a healthy body, it is important to consume a balanced diet and engage in activities and exercise in a balanced way."

DAY 5 DOSE OF FUN

Use play to learn a fact; tug of war is not abstract

MORE MAGIC

Most people don't like to hear about cutting down calories and giving up foods. Be careful with messaging, even to yourself from yourself. It is important not to create a sense of deprivation but to instead focus on balance. Use visual cues or mental imagery (balance scales, tug-of-war, or even a gas tank) to remind yourself of the need to fuel up appropriately to the activity level of each day.

Belldon Colme, Founder of the Nutri-90 system, likes to use the imagery of Legos to help clients understand how food and its components can build a healthy body. If you'd like to listen to an interview I had with Belldon, visit www.kathrynguylay.com/Belldon to get a downloadable interview delivered right to your inbox.

Recipe

• •

Energizing Granola

Ingredients:
- 8 cups rolled oats
- 1 ½ cups chopped pecans
- 1 ½ cups sliced almonds

In separate bowl:
- 1 cup dried cranberries
- 1 cup dried apples, chopped
- 1 cup raisins
- 1 cup dried plums, chopped
- ¼ cup crystallized candied ginger, minced

In a small saucepan:
- ½ cup mild-flavored olive oil
- ½ cup packed brown sugar
- 1 cup honey
- Zest of 2 oranges
- Juice of ½ an orange
- ½ teaspoon salt
- 2 teaspoons cinnamon
- ½ teaspoon cloves

Directions:

Preheat oven to 350 degrees. Line a large rectangular cake pan or two jelly roll pans with parchment paper. Stir the ingredients in the saucepan and heat until the mixture begins to boil. Remove from the heat and pour over the oats, pecans, and almonds. Stir well to combine. Pour oat/nut mixture into prepared pan and bake in preheated oven for 20 minutes, stirring once or twice so the oats and nuts bake evenly and are golden. Once out of the oven, add the dried fruit immediately and mix well. Put into airtight containers and let cool to room temperature before sealing. Granola freezes well. Serve with milk or yogurt, topped with fresh plums or pears or apples.

Day Six

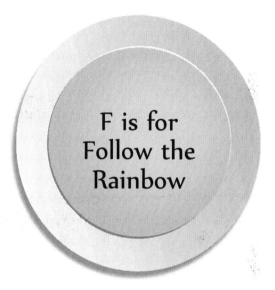

F is for Follow the Rainbow

For my first book, *Mountain Mantras: Wellness and Life Lessons from the Slopes*, I interviewed dozens of Olympic athletes to learn the secrets of their eating practices. I expected to hear complex methods and formulas, given that each athlete generally works with a specialized sports nutritionist. The reality is that Olympians apply concepts that are simple enough for everyone to follow and are, in especially one example, quite fun. That fun guideline is to *follow the rainbow* when choosing fruits and veggies.

In fact, the U.S. Ski Team often adds competitive flair to their mealtimes by seeing who can create the most colorful plate when visiting the salad bar. The minimum goal is to get three colors, but the more the healthier! And this is a competitive bunch.

Foods' natural colors often correlate to certain micronutrients. For example, red is associated with lycopene and heart health. Orange and yellow fruits and vegetables often are loaded with vitamin A, which supports your immune system as well as skin and vision health. Green is associated with folate and other B-vitamins as well as calcium, which is good for your bones and teeth and the digestive and cardiovascular systems. The blue and purple group will assure you a bounty of antioxidants, which support healthy aging. White is associated with potassium and fiber, found in veggies, such as jicama, potatoes, and mushrooms. When you go to the grocery store, challenge yourself (and your kids!) to find different fruits and veggies in various colors.

GIVE IT A GO, EAT A RAINBOW

The concept of eating the rainbow birthed Rainbow Days in schools, a program I have traveled around the country to implement. Kids wear colorful clothes and become ambassadors of a certain color. The kids learn all the different fruits and veggies in a color group, and they eagerly taste different healthy foods across a beautiful arrangement by color. Teachers and parents comment on the exciting positive behavior changes in kids: higher consumption of healthy foods and less pickiness at mealtimes and snack times. But teachers, parents, and kids often asked if there was anything fun I could leave behind to remind them of that fun Rainbow Day.

Thus was born the *Give It a Go, Eat a Rainbow* series, which includes charming illustrations from my then 13-year old son, Alexander, combined with real-life photography to create an augmented reality that immediately draws kids into the story. Kids are introduced to Blake, the main character, who feels sleepy (low energy) and wonders why he doesn't have the energy to play like other kids. Blake, who shrinks down to tiny size, meets a friendly, magical leprechaun who takes Blake on a journey to find the pot of gold (a metaphor for good health and energy).

WHERE DOES A RAINBOW GROW?

Then we met kids who asked, "Why can't I get my rainbow foods in the form of Skittles and Starburst?" Can you just hear the Debbie Downer music in the background: "wah wah wah..."?

Wanting to keep to my rules of not calling food bad (even if they do contain seriously harmful chemicals, like food dyes that are banned in many European countries), I went back to Alexander and said, "Pleeeeease do another book with me about eating the rainbow, this time so that we can teach kids that a healthy rainbow comes from plants, not artificial colors!"

Alexander agreed and created a new character, Sammy the Bunny, who takes Blake on a journey to discover from where healthy, rainbow-colored foods come. In *Where Does a Rainbow Grow?*, the bunny is often peeking out at the reader from various places on the page, eliciting surprise and giggles from kids and parents alike. Laugh your way to good health, I say.

DAY 6 DOSE OF FUN

> *Eat colors from nature or farms,*
> *not diamonds and clovers from Lucky Charms*

MORE MAGIC

How fun would it be to combine the tasks of building literacy, bonding, and establishing healthy habits for life all at once? If you are a parent, you can create this combo platter by simply choosing books for your child that support healthy living. I'd love to invite you to listen to an interview I did with the authors of four children's books, Todd and Jackie Courtney. Their books cover manners, respect and responsibility. Visit www.kathrynguylay.com/ ToddandJackie to get a downloadable interview delivered right to your inbox as well as a digital copy of their children's book, *Be Responsible Like Max*. What fun!

Recipe

Rainbow Smoothie

I have served this delicious smoothie as part of Rainbow Day programming on many occasions. The verdict? Thumbs up!

Ingredients:

- ¼ cup cherries (Red)
- 1 carrot (Orange)
- ½ banana (Yellow)
- 1 handful of spinach (Green)
- ¼ cup blackberries or blueberries (Blue/Purple)
- ½ cup Greek yogurt, vanilla flavor (White)
- 1 teaspoon lemon juice
- 1 teaspoon honey (optional)
- Ice

Directions:

Put ingredients in a blender and add ice/water (about 3-4 ounces) to blend to your desired consistency. Serve immediately. Enjoy!

Day Seven

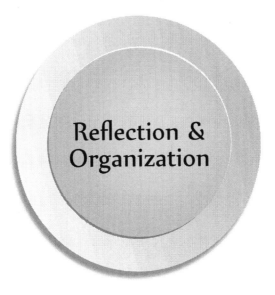

Reflection &
Organization

Day Eight

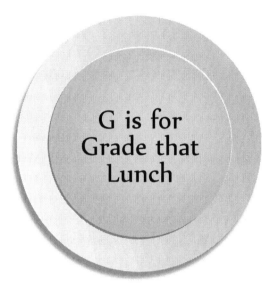

G is for Grade that Lunch

Good news, bad news. Our family had a difficult and memorable transition when we switched from the preschool (Montessori school) lunch program to the public school when Alexander was in Kindergarten.

At Montessori, all the parents sent packed lunches, and no sweets were allowed.

When we signed up for public school, I was pleased to hear that the school had a cafeteria where my kids could get lunch every day. No more packing lunches in the morning! Hooray!

But my smile faded when I received my first statement from the school district:

1/15/09 a la carte brownie ($2), a la carte cookie ($1.50) total $3.50

1/16/09 a la carte brownie ($2), a la carte cookie ($1.50) total $3.50

1/17/09 a la carte brownie ($2), a la carte cookie ($1.50) total $3.50

1/18/09 a la carte brownie ($2), a la carte cookie ($1.50) total $3.50

1/19/09 a la carte brownie ($2), a la carte cookie ($1.50) total $3.50

1/22/09 a la carte brownie ($2), a la carte cookie ($1.50) total $3.50

1/23/09 a la carte brownie ($2), a la carte cookie ($1.50) total $3.50

1/24/09 a la carte brownie ($2), a la carte cookie ($1.50) total $3.50

1/25/09 a la carte brownie ($2), a la carte cookie ($1.50) total $3.50

1/26/09 a la carte brownie ($2), a la carte cookie ($1.50) total $3.50

I tried not to be upset with Alexander as I asked him what he usually did at lunchtime.

"Well, we go through this line and take what we want. Then, there is a checkout lady at the end."

"Did she ever say anything to you about how you were just getting a cookie and a brownie?"

"Um, no," Alexander said.

Whether this was the truth or not, I will never know. But, thanks to my experience as a nutrition educator for kids, I was seasoned to know that punishment and forced action were not the way to go. I needed to figure out a way to empower Alexander to make good decisions on his own.

GRADE THAT LUNCH!

I contacted Alexander's teacher the next morning and asked if I could do a volunteer nutrition lesson in his grade the following week.

"Sure!" she said. "I have been wanting to do something about the quality of my kids' lunches. In the afternoon, I can tell the difference between who's had a good lunch and who hasn't."

So I showed up with the game: Grade That Lunch.

"I'm going to show you a series of lunch boxes, and you will give each lunch a score. Each food group included gets a point. The highest score possible is a five. You get one point for having each of the following: whole grain, protein, dairy/calcium, fruits, and veggies. Are you ready?"

"*Yes!*"

So I put up the first picture of a lunch.

Lunch menu example #1:

- French fries and ketchup

- Power drink or soda
- Candy bar

There was a pause as the kids tried to reconcile the food groups with the picture. A little girl raised her hand. "Is it possible to get a zero?"

"Yes! That's right. This lunch is a *zero*." Then we moved on to the next picture.

Lunch menu example #2:

- Hamburger on white bun
- Tater tots and ketchup
- Chocolate chip cookie
- Sweetened iced tea

The kids studied the photo.

"One?"

"You got it. We can count the hamburger meat as protein. Harvard's Healthy Eating Plate mentions that white potatoes don't count as a veggie, and the fried aspect of the tater tots renders them unhealthy. Let's move on to another lunch!"

Lunch menu example #3:

- Enriched crackers
- Cheese and ham

- Reese's Peanut Butter Cup
- Sour candies

"I think a two," a voice came from the back of the room.

"Yes, we are moving up," I responded.

The meat on the picture was not particularly appetizing, but we decided to count it as protein. The cheese earned a point for dairy.

"What about a point for the crackers as whole grains?" another voice questioned.

"Nope. The word 'enriched' gives away the fact that the grains have been processed and are no longer whole. Let's move on."

Lunch menu example #4:

- Tuna salad on enriched bread
- Cherry tomatoes and cucumbers
- Clementine
- Pretzels
- Pickles
- Cake

"Hmmm," I heard.

"I think we are moving up to a three. I see a fruit, veggies, and protein," said a child in the first row.

"How could you make this lunch even better?"

We brainstormed and decided that exchanging the enriched bread with whole grain bread would be good. We could also omit the pretzels or forgo the cake and have the clementine for dessert.

I noticed Alexander taking in all of the discussion among his classmates, despite not saying anything himself. He was hearing from his friends what a *cool* lunch was.

Lunch menu example #5:

- Chicken salad in whole-wheat pita
- Red pepper, carrots, hummus
- Greek yogurt and fresh berries
- Whole-grain/veggie pasta salad

"*FIVE! FIVE!*" The kids were all now really excited and were shouting.

"I see chicken for protein! Hummus, too!"

"Whole grains in the pita! Calcium in the Greek yogurt!"

"Fruits *and* veggies!"

The teacher helped me to calm the class. Then, we talked about how delicious the *five* lunch looked.

A few weeks later, Alexander's teacher called me with good news and bad news.

"The good news is that the kids' lunches are improving a ton. I'm seeing a noticeable change in attention and attitude after lunch. Thank you, Kathryn."

"You're welcome. What's the bad news?"

"Well, the principal had to intervene in the lunchroom a few times these last two weeks. He had heard tons of noise and wanted to know why there were numbers being screamed from the lunchroom and echoing down the halls."

"What was going on?"

"I think the kids just got a little overexcited about being able to assign their *own grades* at school."

DAY 8 DOSE OF FUN

It's okay to yell and shout;
if a great lunch is what you're excited about

MORE MAGIC

Alexander's lunches started to steadily improve after the *Grade That Lunch* game. Can you guess what the key ingredients were for the game's success? There are three: Educate, Inspire, and Give

Choice. The more you can take the struggle out of nutrition and food and replace it with education, inspiration, and choice, the more fun you will have.

If you'd like to listen to another story from a mom that was able to affect her child's nutrition program at school in a positive way, I invite you to listen to an interview with the co-founder of Nourish Schools, Katherine Sumner. Visit www.kathrynguylay.com/Katherine to get a downloadable interview delivered right to your inbox.

Recipe

● ●

Fiesta Casserole

This lunch recipe won the Healthy Kids Lunchtime Challenge State Dinner and secured my daughter and my entry to the White House to meet Michelle Obama. What an honor!

Ingredients:

- 1 cup brown rice
- 1 ½ cups quinoa, rinsed
- 2 (16 ounce) jars of your favorite salsa
- 4 (15 ounce) cans of assorted beans, rinsed and drained
- 2 (16 ounce) containers of cottage cheese
- Juice of 2 limes
- 2 teaspoons chili powder
- 2 teaspoons ground cumin
- 1 bunch fresh cilantro, coarsely chopped
- 8 ounces of shredded cheese of your choice (we like the Mexican blend for this recipe)
- Salt to taste

For serving:

- Sliced carrots, celery, jicama and avocado

Directions:

Preheat oven to 350 degrees. In two saucepans, cook the rice and quinoa according to the package directions. Alternatively, read Day 20 and cook the rice and quinoa in rice cookers. In a very large bowl, combine the cooked rice, quinoa, salsa, beans, cottage cheese, lime juice, chili powder, cumin, and cilantro. Spread the mixture in two (9 x 12) baking dishes, cover with foil, and bake until the rice and quinoa are light brown, about 40 minutes. Carefully remove the foil from both pans and sprinkle the cheese on top of each casserole. Return to oven and bake until the cheese is melted and bubbling, about five minutes. Season to taste with salt and serve with sliced veggies.

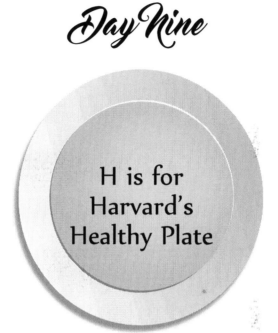

Day Nine

H is for Harvard's Healthy Plate

How did we survive the plague of the pyramids? I have been in the nutrition education field long enough to consider myself a survivor of the Food Pyramids, the diabetes-inducing diagrams from the 1980s and 90s that led people to eat bread by the loaf and low-fat cookies by the bag. Thank goodness for Michelle Obama and her efforts to create a healthy and easy-to-understand visual aid to illustrate nutritional guidelines.

Yes, MyPlate was a huge step in the right direction. MyPlate is a nutritional icon that I'm happy to see on the walls of school lunchrooms. Keeping it simple, here are the key take-aways that Nurture teaches with MyPlate:

- Make half of your plate fruits and veggies, with an emphasis on the veggies!

- Eat lean protein. My dad (Dr. Bob)'s rule for breakfast applies to every snack and meal throughout the day.

- Make your grains whole grains. While MyPlate asks for only half your grains to be whole, I recommend avoiding processed grains whenever possible.

- Choose your beverage wisely. You know the saying "You are what you eat." But our diabetes issues nationally are also very much related to what we drink. Cut out the soda and sugary drinks. Kids should not have more than one cup of fruit juice a day (or better yet, none). And no large sodas, please.

Harvard's Healthy Plate takes MyPlate's positive momentum a step further. This adaptation of MyPlate highlights water, not dairy, as the beverage of choice. I also appreciate the addition of the healthy oils on the side. There are a few other differences as well, but both are far better than the disastrous food pyramid.

Warning to folks in Idaho: Harvard's Healthy Plate does not count potatoes as veggies. I hope folks in the "potato state" can forgive

Harvard, just as we have overlooked Dan Quayle's misspelling of our plural veggie and carbohydrate.

DAY 9 DOSE OF FUN

Choose Harvard's Healthy Plate or MyPlate
for advice that makes you feel great

MORE MAGIC

Unlike the pyramid, the plate model is actionable and applicable to meals and everyday life. Engage your creative side by downloading a color-in worksheet of a plate and draw your favorite meal. Color code if you want to take it a step further. Get your own color-in plates by visiting www.kathrynguylay.com/plates.

Recipe

• •

Colorful Quinoa Salad

This recipe should get the thumbs up from the folks at Harvard. No potatoes.

Ingredients:

- 2 cups quinoa
- 2 tablespoon lemon juice
- 1 red bell pepper, diced
- 1 yellow bell pepper, diced
- 1 cucumber, diced
- ⅓ of a red onion, diced
- ⅓ jar of roasted bell peppers, diced
- 4 to 8 ounces of Feta cheese (depends on how much you like cheese!)

For dressing:

- Salt and pepper to taste
- ¼ cup extra virgin olive oil
- ⅛ cup balsamic vinegar
- Juice from one lemon
- Fresh herbs (I suggest ½ bunch parsley, washed

and chopped, and some washed and snipped mint leaves)

Directions:

Rinse quinoa well. (Quinoa can have a coating of bitter-tasting saponins that you want to be sure to remove). For easier digestion, you can soak your grains: leave grains covered with non-chlorinated water, plus an acidic medium, for about 7-8 hours. The amount of acidic medium is 1 tablespoon for every 1 cup of grains. Your best choices for an acidic medium are lemon juice or vinegar. Quinoa is one of the easier grains to digest (along with amaranth, brown rice, buckwheat, and millet) because it contains less phytates than other grains.

Cook the quinoa on the stovetop or in a rice cooker. In a bowl, mix the cooked quinoa with all of the other ingredients except for the cheese, and stir to combine. Serve with feta sprinkled over the top. Enjoy!

Day Ten

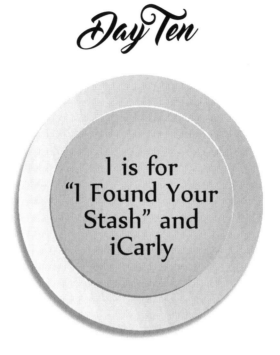

1 is for
"I Found Your
Stash" and
iCarly

In the bottom of Elena's dresser drawer, during spring cleanout, I found a huge stash of all of the candies I had told our kids to avoid: jelly beans, gummy bears, sticky lollipops, and everything with the banned-in-Europe chemicals I mentioned on Day 6 (Follow the Rainbow).

How many years worth of Halloween candy was stashed here!?

It was a huge stash.

I had been preaching to the kids about the dangers of food coloring, but I had been using terms they not only didn't know but also couldn't care less about.

"Some food additives are actually neurotoxins!"

"The yellow food dye Tartrazine has been banned in France, Germany, and many other places; but our country still uses it!"

"I read today that food dyes might be linked to the increase in Attention Deficit Disorder!"

I looked down at the cesspool of food coloring in Elena's drawer. At that moment, she walked into the room.

"That's *mine!*" she screamed, pointing to the drawer.

These chemical-laden candies had become valuable commodities to my daughter. I knew that being the *candy police* would make matters even worse, so I tried out *candy lawyer* and started negotiations.

"I know you really want to watch iCarly, and I won't let you," I said in as calm a voice as I could muster. iCarly is a show on Nickelodeon that is most appropriate for teens and tweens, but my fourth grade daughter was intent on being a little precocious.

"Yes," Elena said suspiciously.

"I'll buy this candy from you. A nickel for a small one and a dime for a big one. I bet you have almost enough to barter for a few shows of iCarly. Each show will cost you a dollar."

"A *quarter* for the big ones," Elena countered, and we made a deal.

And Elena got to watch nearly an entire season of iCarly. I mentioned it was a pretty sizable stash. We actually had fun watching it together, and I especially loved the character of Carly's brother, Spencer. It ended up being fun and good bonding time that both of us will cherish forever.

DAY 10 DOSE OF FUN

Learn to let go. Let your kids watch the iCarly show

MORE MAGIC

I'm not suggesting that you indulge your kids in TV or bribe them at every turn. I do suggest, however, that you figure out what currency is most important to you, your kids, and anyone you love. Especially with kids, it is key to know if they value academic performance, sports, or simply special privileges, such as TV or outings. Then, when you need some leverage, pull out the card that they value the most and make an agreement or compromise. Making nutrition fun is about keeping your relationships positive and supportive, and the anti-fun dynamic is one where parties have locked-horns with no room to breathe.

If you'd like more details about how to communicate with kids in a positive way about nutrition and food, I'll direct you to an interview I had with Jed Doherty of the *We Choose Respect* podcast. Visit www.kathrynguylay.com/WeChooseRespect to get the interview delivered right to your inbox.

Day Eleven

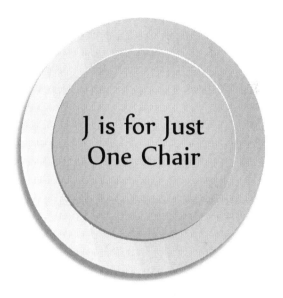

J is for Just One Chair

"Just a table for two," Valla, a friend of ours, said with a bit of disgust as he, Jeff, and I walked into a restaurant in the heart of downtown Chicago. It was a busy night. The hostess looked at our group of *three* with suspicion.

"Just *ugh*. These guys are newlyweds. They can sit on each other's laps."

"Excuse me?" said the hostess.

"It's ridiculous. When they speak to each other, all I hear is 'smootchy whooshey,'" Valla continued. "It's really annoying. But trust me, they'll share a chair. And probably a meal, too."

The hostess was still looking at him with confusion. Valla was a medical student in one of his rotations at a Chicago hospital. Rather than get his own apartment for his short three-month stint in town, he had asked if he could stay in our living room on Lake Shore Drive.

"Of course, Dr. Valla," we told him. "Just as long as you don't mind being the third wheel." Valla knew us well enough to know what he was getting into.

The hostess led us to a table in the corner.

"Seriously," Valla said to her. "Just count them as one person. They will certainly eat off the same plate."

That was indeed true. Jeff and I loved to go out to dinner every Friday night, but we had learned over time that eating an entire entrée each was simply too much, so we always picked one to share.

It was my turn to order. "We'll have the herb crusted ..."

"...Salmon, please," finished Jeff.

I smiled at Jeff in agreement. As much as our finishing each other's sentences annoyed Valla, he conceded the point that restaurant portions had ballooned way out of control. He had heard a story about how the Center for Science in the Public Interest had recently started including a section in its newsletter called "Food Porn."

"Finally, we doctors are starting to pay attention," said Valla, as he smiled and eyed the table of six women next to us on a girls' night out.

"Food porn! What does *that* mean?" I said too loudly.

"They are comparing what the food industry is doing, like how some companies are creating packaging for snacking in reasonable portions. Then, on the same page, they show some really outrageous stuff. They call that the *food porn*."

At the mention of porn, several of the girls at the nearby table looked over. Valla was really good-looking, the tall, dark, and mysterious type.

"Can you give me an example of food porn?" asked Jeff, interrupting Valla's stare at the other table.

"The magazine article picks out a food item or entrée that goes beyond the limits of acceptable societal norms," Valla said. "Having 2,000 calories per serving, three days' worth of saturated fat, or a week's worth of sodium. It's fascinating, yet a bit disgusting at the same time."

Our food arrived, and we were about to settle in. Jeff and I decided to share a fork.

"You know what, guys? I'm outta here," Valla said.

Then, to the many giggles of the table beside us, Valla abandoned us and joined the girls-night-out-table. We didn't see him until the next day.

PORTION DISTORTION OVER TIME

Several generations ago, it might not have been as critical for us to follow a rule such as splitting an entrée when dining out. Portion distortion is a relatively new phenomenon in the food industry, and it is critical for your health that you understand the implications of the changes in portion size over time.

When McDonald's first opened in 1955, it offered one drink size: 6.5 ounces. Today, the kids' size is 12 ounces, and the large is 32 ounces! As you may know, choosing soda as a beverage is not an optimal choice; but what if you do decide to have a soda once in awhile? What are the implications of having one of today's large sodas as compared to 1955's 6.5-ounce serving?

The difference is an extra 245 calories and 17.5 teaspoons of sugar! To burn the extra calories in a single large soda would take nearly an hour of biking.

Michael Bloomberg, the former mayor of New York City, didn't think all the soda drinkers out there would burn the additional calories with physical activity. Concerned about the growing costs of diabetes and other nutrition-related diseases, he proposed limits on the sale of sugary drinks in an effort to keep servings to 16 ounces or less. Unfortunately, his proposal was overturned.

What about bagels? In the past 40 years, bagels have nearly doubled in size. The three-inch diameter bagels that I remember as a kid had about 140 calories, much fewer than the 350 calories in the six-inch bagels you often find at stores today.

The calorie difference between the bagel of the 1970s and a bagel of today is about 210 calories, and most of that comes from processed grains that will turn from sugar to fat in your body unless you burn it off first. In other words, you'd better be running those two miles to the bagel shop—assuming you want to stay as svelte as the '70s disco stars.

SERVING SIZE DOES NOT EQUAL PORTION SIZE

A critical first step is to understand the difference between a *serving size* and a *portion size*. A serving size is a specified amount shown on the Nutrition Facts label on a package. The information there, including the number of calories, applies to the serving size.

A portion is how much you actually eat or drink in one sitting; it is also the amount of food you get in a single restaurant order. Guess what? On average, one portion size is equal to two or three serving sizes. Food packaging is tricky, and most people don't do the math to realize how many calories they are actually consuming. Shoppers might see 250 calories per serving on the Nutrition Facts label but end up eating the entire box or bag in one sitting. They forget to multiply the number of calories by the number of servings. If there are two servings in the package, they've just eaten 500 calories, not 250. When reading a Nutrition Facts label, before you read any of the other information, always start by looking at the number of servings.

Once you know the difference between the amount of food in a serving and the amount in a portion, you can use strategies to control the size of your portions. We've already discussed sharing an entrée at a restaurant. If you don't have anyone to share with, simply ask your waiter to save half of your entrée in a to-go bag and have it for lunch the following day. At home, use a 9-inch plate instead of a 12-inch plate. The visual cue of a full plate, even one that's smaller, can lead to satisfaction. Don't eat directly from the box or bag. Pour a serving onto a plate and put the container away. Finally, use a comparison to everyday objects to get a sense of what a reasonable portion size is. I have never weighed my food, nor do I count grams or calories on a daily basis. I control my portions by understanding what is a reasonable amount of food to add to my plate. Here are the guidelines I follow:

- Carbohydrates. Amount: 1⁄2 cup cooked, about the size of half a baseball.

- Protein. Amount: 3 ounces, about the size of a deck of cards.

- Dairy. Amount: 1 ounce, about the size of four dice. Nut butter. Amount: 1 tablespoon, about the size of half a ping-pong ball.

- Oils and dressings. Amount: 2 tablespoons, about the size of one ping-pong ball.

- Vegetables. Amount: Unlimited, pile them up without worrying about quantities!

DAY 11 DOSE OF FUN

Size food as a ball or card deck, to keep portion sizes in check

MORE MAGIC

Ballooning portion sizes are a big reason behind our nation's diabetes epidemic. I was amazed to hear the story of Denise Pancryz, now a diabetes reversal expert, who went from having to give herself several shots of insulin every day to being completely drug free thanks to changes in her eating habits. If you'd like to listen to her story yourself, please visit www.kathrynguylay.com/Denise to get our interview delivered right to your inbox.

Day Twelve

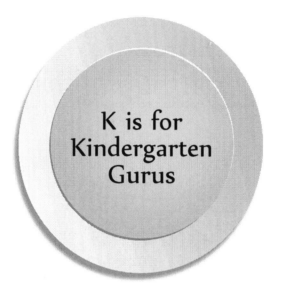

K is for Kindergarten Gurus

Kindergarteners really do know best. Most of us have heard about the book by Robert Fulghum, *All I Really Need to Know I Learned In Kindergarten*. I'd add that these little buggers really know their stuff when it comes to making nutrition fun.

I have learned through my work with tens of thousands of people that, in our American culture, we need to develop a better relationship with food. Eating from fear or guilt is not good for you. Eating to cover up insecure or sad feelings is not good for you, either. In our Make Nutrition Fun Introductory Course, Registered Dietitian Juliette Britton and I help you to identify your "food feeling" and strategies to make nutrition fun with your food feelings in mind. Learn more about this course and others at www.MakeNutritionFun.com. If you deny yourself food, that behavior is equally unhealthy. Recognize, instead, the necessity of food as the gas in our tanks and a source of our energy.

We all need to view food as energy.

The little gurus in a kindergarten classroom drove home that point for me during a lesson that Juliette and I gave at a school in the suburbs of Chicago. The lesson was called *go vs. slow-down* and was designed to avoid confusing nutrition jargon. Keeping it simple allowed us to establish a vocabulary to talk about food in a way that makes sense to kids and refers to what they want to do.

Do they care that canned frosting has fats that may be bad for their hearts? Not so much. Do they care if eating unhealthy foods will make them slow down, not have sustained energy, or make them sleepy? Yes!

By understanding why the body needs food, it becomes much easier to decipher what types of food provide the best fuel. Any food with calories provides energy for the body. However, not all calories are created equal. A powdered-sugar donut has the same number of calories as a bowl of oatmeal with strawberries and slivered almonds. Yet, while the body feels hungry several hours after eating the donut, the oatmeal is filling and nutritious and gives longstanding energy.

So we kicked off the lesson as the kids gathered around us on the reading rug, many on their knees leaning forward and most struggling not to squirm.

"What foods give the body long-lasting energy?" Juliette asked the eager group of kindergarteners.

"Carrots!"

"Apples!"

"Meat!"

"Cheese!"

"Strawberries!"

"Broccoli!"

These answers are right on target. Note the absence of low-fat energy bars, fast food, baked chips, and processed foods. The only responses were whole foods, mainly fruits and vegetables, which we call *go* foods because they fuel the body with long-lasting energy, vitamins, minerals, and nutrients to support growth and activity. *Go* foods include fruits and vegetables, lean proteins, nuts, legumes, eggs, milk, and whole grains. *Go* foods fuel the body so it can move!

"What foods slow the body down?" I asked the group.

"Cookies!"

"Cake!"

"Ice cream!"

"Brownies!"

"Potato chips!"

"French fries!"

"Candy!"

"Soda!"

These foods have little nutritional value, so we call them *slow-down* foods or *sleepy* foods. These foods may provide a short burst of energy, but they soon leave the body feeling hungry or tired. *Slow-down* foods slow down the body.

"If *slow-down* foods make us sleepy, does that mean we can never eat them?" we asked the kindergarteners.

"No," they say wisely. "*Slow-down* foods are okay every once in awhile."

Whether or not these kindergarten gurus know what the word moderation means, they get the idea that *go* foods are the best, but *slow-down* foods can be part of a balanced diet, when consumed in moderation.

By promoting a balanced and positive relationship with food, we are setting the stage for a healthy, energized relationship with food. Energy is a buzzword loved by kids and adults alike, because it implies movement and fun. *Go* foods, on the one hand, capture this liveliness. *Slow-down* foods, on the other hand, promote sleepiness. And not many children want to feel sleepy!

DAY 12 DOSE OF FUN

Begin to view food as fuel,
like the Kindergarten Gurus teach at school

MORE MAGIC

Today, I'd like for you to start using a new vocabulary around food that takes the charge out of the situation. Can you experiment with removing bad and other negative words from mealtimes, shopping, and discussions around food? If the go and slow-down words don't resonate with you, perhaps a traffic light (green, yellow, red) might work instead. Experiment with simple word changes and see how the energy shifts in your kitchen and at the dinner table.

If you'd like to learn more about programs that teach kids about healthy eating in a positive way, I invite you to listen to an interview I did with Registered Dietitian Laurie McBride. We talked about a program for high-BMI kids based on fun and fellowship.

Visit www.kathrynguylay.com/Laurie to get a downloadable interview delivered right to your inbox.

Day Thirteen

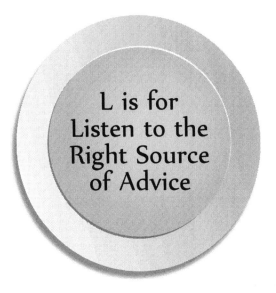

L is for Listen to the Right Source of Advice

Lately, we've had a lot of mixed signals about what we're supposed to be eating. Nutritional advice, in an official form—beyond what parents or grandparents teach about healthy eating—has been around for just over a century. The U.S. Department of Agriculture (USDA) published its first nutrition guidelines in 1894. These guidelines originated as a simple farmers' bulletin, but the advice continued to grow from there. What is most confusing to me about how that advice evolved over the 20th century is that, even as the problem being addressed changed so dramatically, our nation did not consider that we might need to change the source of our advice. In the first half of the last century, which included the Great Depression and two World Wars, the problem was that we simply did not have enough food. One of the primary reasons soldiers were turned away from military service was because they were malnourished. The National School Lunch Program, also run by the USDA, began in 1946 as a way to reach children who might otherwise not have access to adequate nutrition. Involving the Department of Agriculture at this point, when the focus was addressing inadequate nutrition, made perfect sense.

As the 20th century came to a close, however, the problem was no longer one of adequate calories. In 2005, the *New England Journal of Medicine* reported that, for the first time in American history, today's children may have a shorter average lifespan than their parents due to the health-related impact of obesity and nutritionally-linked diseases. The problem has shifted so dramatically that more soldiers are now turned away from military service for being overweight than underweight. Health care costs have skyrocketed into the trillions of dollars to address nutritionally related diseases. The crazy thing is that food insecurity and malnutrition still exist! Thanks to the USDA, we have a flood of corn and starchy products in our food system, providing plenty of calories while lacking nutritional balance. Because starchy foods are plentiful and cheap, the lower-income population is disproportionately affected by obesity. Food distribution lines across the nation are full of the malnourished and overfed.

TIME FOR A NEW VOICE

Let's say that your car doesn't seem to be working well. It is sputtering and clanking and doesn't seem safe to drive. You have always brought it to your favorite mechanic because he seems to understand how to fix whatever mechanical problem might be at play. He has his standard set of tools, and he loves to use them. You hesitate going back this time, however, because you have a sense that the problem has nothing to do with the car itself but instead with the gas that you are putting into it. You've always bought your gas from that same favorite mechanic because it's what he recommends. So, where do you go now?

The USDA is the old-school mechanic. The standard tools are its subsidy programs. Who is the broken down car in this metaphor? You! Your kids! Your friends and family! If you are interested in learning more about the USDA and its role in the food chain, I encourage you to watch *Fed Up*, the 2014 documentary by executive producers Katie Couric and Laurie David.

Based on the sad state of American wellness, it's clear that the federal government is no longer the best source of information and guidance.

Who should fill the void? I suggest turning to nutritional experts that are heart-centered and take an individualized approach. Avoid the "my way or the highway" teachers that only promote a supplemental program or product from which they stand to gain financially.

DAY 13 DOSE OF FUN

Don't roll the dice, double-check your advice

MORE MAGIC

The Make Nutrition Fun Summit includes interviews with dozens of heart-centered nutrition experts who will uplift you and provide actionable advice. Find out more about the Summit (which you can listen to as you're out for walks with your dogs, kids, or in solitude) and combine education with physical activity. More information can be found at www.makenutritionfun.com/summit.

Recipe

- -

Minestrone Soup

Ingredients:

- 6 cups chicken broth
- 1 can cannellini beans, drained and rinsed
- 1 can (28 ounces) diced tomatoes
- 2 tablespoons olive oil
- 2 yellow onions, chopped fine
- 4 garlic cloves, minced
- ½ cup dry pasta – Orzo and Ditalini work well
  – Gluten free also can be used
- 1 bag frozen veggies – look for an Italian blend
- ¼ cup minced fresh basil
- ½ cup Parmesan cheese
- Salt and pepper to taste

Directions:

Bring broth, beans, and tomatoes to a boil in a large pot. Meanwhile, sauté onions until shimmering. Add garlic and add to boiling mixture. Add pasta and cook for 10 minutes. Stir in veggies and basil and cook for another two minutes. Season with salt and pepper. Serve with Parmesan cheese and a drizzle of olive oil. Serves 6.

Day Fourteen

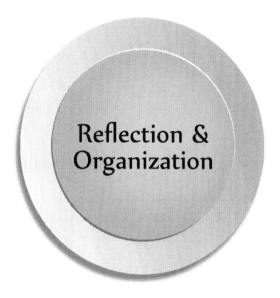

Reflection &
Organization

Day Fifteen

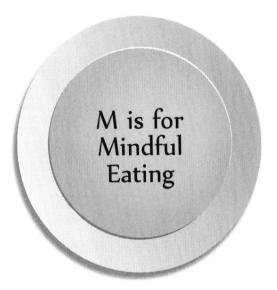

M is for
Mindful
Eating

Many of us sit down with a bag of chips while in front of the TV, only to realize that our hand is scraping around in the salty crumbs at the bottom of the bag before we've ever really tasted our snack.

What? Did I eat the entire thing already?

Anyone that multi-tasks with eating (working and eating, watching TV and eating, driving and eating, the list goes on) knows this experience well.

So, I was thrilled when I had the opportunity to interview mindfulness eating expert Charlotte Hammond (R.D.) on my podcast *Mountain Mantras: Wellness and Life Lessons*. In this 45-minute discussion, we uncovered three steps that will allow you to immediately bring more mindfulness into your eating.

Step 1: Breathe between bites

Step 2: Play with your food; get all your senses involved

Step 3: Take your time: 20 minutes is needed on average for your stomach to send a signal to your brain that you are full

Charlotte also offered important advice for teens, a population she focuses on in her work. Top tips for teens include:

1) Get sugar out of the liquids you consume

2) Focus on foods you can HAVE (not forbidden foods), and

3) Reframe our vocabulary around food to focus on quality: 50% of meals should be low starch

For families, Charlotte recommends that you study your food bills so that you can better understand, in a mindful way, where can you save and where can you splurge. Areas she recommends for a splurge include clean eating to avoid the most harmful pesticides in produce. An easy way to remember which produce you might want to splurge on for organic is the ABC method. A for Apples, B for Berries, and C for Celery (plus anything with leaves).

To listen to my interview with Charlotte, please visit <u>www.</u><u>kathrynguylay.com/Charlotte</u> to get a downloadable interview delivered right to your inbox.

DAY 15 DOSE OF FUN

> *Eating should never be a race, slow down and enjoy the pace*

MORE MAGIC

I'm going to assign you a simple yet powerful exercise to allow you to incorporate more mindfulness into your eating. It's called the raisin exercise:

- Give yourself about five minutes to complete the exercise. No rushing!
- Get a raisin and put it in the palm of your hand. Start by just observing its visual qualities. Is it shiny or dull? Is it smooth or wrinkly?
- Then really feel the raisin. Roll it between your fingers and observe its texture. Hard or soft? Sticky or smushy?
- Now, close your eyes and put the raisin in your mouth. First let it sit on your tongue without chewing.
- When you begin chewing, bite slowing and extend the amount of time it takes to chew. What does the raisin

taste like as it moves between your teeth and around your mouth? Do you feel the urge to swallow right away? Try to hold off on that urge for just a few moments. Then go ahead and swallow the raisin.

As you move through your day and its meals and snacks, see if you can appreciate the sensual qualities of your food. Is your appreciation for your food growing?

If you'd like to listen to more from mindfulness experts, allow me to suggest the following interviews I've conducted with parents and experts on this topic. Visit the links below to get downloadable interviews delivered right to your inbox:

- My interview with Mira Binzen, who has taught yoga and mindfulness to children since 2002, is available at www.kathrynguylay.com/Mira.
- Ryan Redman is a mindfulness expert and the Executive Director of the Flourish Foundation. Our conversation is available at www.kathrynguylay.com/Ryan.
- My interview with Annie Mahon, author of *Things I Did When I Was Hangry*, is available at www.kathrynguylay.com/Annie.

Day Sixteen

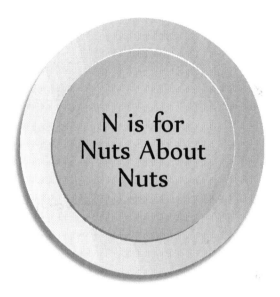

N is for
Nuts About
Nuts

Nutrition lessons on a Friday afternoon? I knew when I got the call from the fifth grade teacher to schedule the nutrition lesson that I would have to be creative and engaging to keep the students' attention.

My task? Educate these students, who couldn't wait to get started on their weekend activities, about the importance of and difference between the three macronutrients: carbohydrates, fats, and protein.

Most of the kids were looking out the window at the beautiful day awaiting them...until I started running around the room.

"I'm really active! I need fast-acting fuel! Give me carbohydrates!" Then, I pretended to reach into my pocket for a snack. "Oooh! An almond! Almonds are nuts, which have carbohydrates."

Then I started to pretend to lift weights. I was squatting down and pulling up with my imaginary weights. As I groaned and grunted, the kids started to really pay attention. And laugh at me.

"Phew! Now that I'm done with that, I need to rebuild my muscles! I need protein!"

So I pretended to reach into my pocket again. "Oooh! A cashew! Cashews are nuts, which have protein."

Then I rubbed my tummy. "I'm still hungry. What macronutrient besides protein really helps me feel satisfied?" I pretended to reach into my pocket again. "Oooh! A macadamia. Macadamias are nuts, which have healthy fat. Healthy fat makes you feel full and helps your body at the cellular level."

I went on to explain that nuts are an example of a balanced food that contains all three of the macronutrients. Then I talked about the foods that are heavier on carbohydrates (grains, fruits, and veggies), heavier on fats (olive oil, coconut oil) and heavier on proteins (meat, poultry, and fish). To keep the kids' attention, I continued to run around the room, tapping the kids to test them on macronutrients.

"Name a food that has protein!"

Steak, lentils, beans.

"Name a food that has fat!"

Olive oil, butter, cheese.

"Name a food that has carbohydrates!"

Crackers, apples, rice.

At the end of the school year, I asked the students which lesson was their favorite.

"The one where you ran around the class like a crazy lady, talking about nuts!" one student said.

Another added, "Mrs. Guylay, we love when you come to teach in our class, even though you are a bit nuts."

DAY 16 DOSE OF FUN

Make healthy choices and follow your gut,
even if everyone thinks you're a nut

MORE MAGIC

We've already talked about food groups (On Day 8, Grade That Lunch), but having a basic understanding of the three macronutrients can also help you and your kids keep things in balance. Most Americans get too many carbohydrates, and our fat-phobic culture has overly reduced our intake of healthy fats, such as oils and omega-3 fatty acids. Remember that our brains absolutely love fatty acids, and our skin, hair, nails, and eyes shine when we get enough healthy fats. Even if it is for vanity's sake, make healthy fats your friend.

For those that want to increase their knowledge about nutrition and get into the details of macronutrients and micronutrients, I love Dr. Meaghan Kirshling's podcast *Beyond the Basics Health Academy*. I was honored to be her guest on episode 123, during which we talked about healthy eating habits for kids. You can listen to our interview at www.beyondthebasicshealthacademy.com/podcast-123/.

Recipe

Pumpkin Pecan Oatmeal

I urge you to read the rice cooker instructions (Day 20), as this recipe is so easy with a rice cooker. You can use the stovetop, too. A wonderful warming way to start your day, especially in the Fall or Winter.

Ingredients:
- 1 cup old fashioned oats or steel cut oats
- ¼ cup packed brown sugar
- 1 teaspoon pumpkin pie spice
- pinch of salt
- 1 cup milk
- ½ cup canned pumpkin
- 1 egg
- 3 tablespoons chopped pecans

Directions (using a rice cooker):

Combine oats, brown sugar, pumpkin pie spice, and pinch of salt in rice cooker. Whisk milk, pumpkin and egg in small bowl. Pour over oat mixture; stir to combine. Cover and press down the "on" button.

Button will click up to the "warm" setting when oats are done, about 20 minutes. Unplug cooker. Serve topped with pecans and an extra splash of milk, if desired.

Day Seventeen

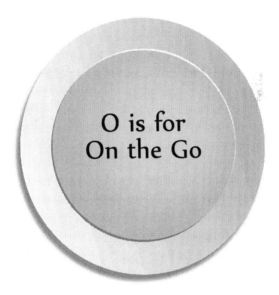

O is for
On the Go

Over the years, I've learned strategies to help with the running-out-the-door dynamic.

In our busy and fast paced lives, we might intellectually know how important it is to eat healthy meals and snacks, yet sometimes we just don't make the time for it.

I can be a drill sergeant when trying to get my kids out the door in the morning. These frantic moments are usually when we and our kids grab for the processed energy bar. We might even stop at a drive-through to quell the hunger pains and stop the complaining!

Here's a short list that will help you make better choices, even under time pressure:

- Make healthy choices available by putting grab-and-go items in your refrigerator and at eye level on your shelves (think sandwiches, wraps, and even brown bag meals).
- In the evenings, cut up fruits and vegetables so that they are already in containers that can be grabbed in seconds.
- Portion out dipping sauces in small containers to accompany cut-up veggies and fruits or even sandwiches. Dips increase the fun factor for most foods.
- Use a rice cooker (coming up on Day 20) to make a hot breakfast pot that folks can dip a spoon into to start their breakfast bar (explained on Day 2, Break the Fast, Not Your Tooth)

DAY 17 DOSE OF FUN

Don't worry if you're on the go, bring your healthy food in tow

MORE MAGIC

When I interviewed Janette Hillis-Jaffe, wellness coach, speaker, and author of *Everyday Healing, Stand Up, Take Charge, and Get Your Health Back...One Day at a Time,* she shared some great tips on eating on the go, even when you're traveling to several cities in a week. Janette experienced this challenge on her extensive book tour and mastered the art of healthy living, even out of hotel rooms. Her tips include avoiding room service and instead going to local grocery stores for easy to assemble meals, consisting of fruits, veggies, canned garbanzos, and other legumes. Listening to her advice reminded me that we often use travel as an excuse for not eating well, when if we simply make it a priority, healthy meals are absolutely within our reach. If you would like to listen to my interview with Janette, please visit www.kathrynguylay. com/Janette to get a downloadable interview delivered right to your inbox.

Day Eighteen

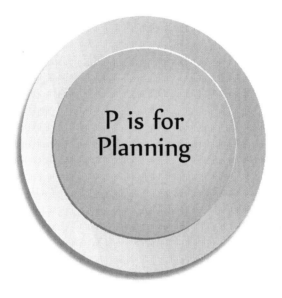

P is for
Planning

Predictable phases in life are few and far between. Around your late 20s and early 30s, however, it is common to feel that you've gone into full *wedding mode*. Attending dozens of weddings a year seems normal. It was 1998 when this phase of life hit Jeff and me, and we needed to plan for a particular wedding in Minneapolis. The groom and dear friend of mine, John, and I met when we had commuted from our respective parents' homes in the suburbs for summer internships in between our sophomore and junior years of college. John was hilarious and smart, attending

Colgate as an English major, so I always tried to use my best SAT words as we rode the train to work with *alacrity*. I didn't know much about John's fiancée, Jen, except that she was very pretty and seemed to have a great sense of humor.

I wouldn't have missed John's wedding for the world, but Jeff and I were working on tough projects with looming deadlines, so we were delayed at our offices. We finally got on the road just six hours before the wedding—with a six-hour drive ahead of us.

We arrived just in time, having driven the entire way with the top of the convertible down in the blazing sun. In our haste (and youth), we had forgotten to put on sunscreen, so when I pulled off my tank top to change into my formal strapless dress, there was a very obvious white seat belt mark in the middle of my sunburn. Our hair was standing on end, and we hadn't eaten anything since morning.

"It's a wedding," Jeff assured me. "There will be tons of food."

So we sat patiently through the ceremony with our tummies grumbling, as we patted down our hair. When we arrived at the reception hall, we strategically waited—like tigers perched high on the savannah—outside the door where the waiters were coming out with finger foods.

"There goes a plate of food!" I yelled, as Jeff went off for an interception. He came back with a puzzled look on his face.

"Mushrooms stuffed with Spam. I didn't think you'd want one."

"Weird. Here's another waiter!" And I went in for the kill.

Spam on a stick?

This Spam surprise happened again and again, as the oddest concoctions of Spam made their way by our salivating mouths. But we just couldn't get into the idea of Spam.

At dinner, we learned that Jen was somehow related to the Spam empire. On the dinner menu? Spam. And Spam.

I ate my side of carrots (with Spam) along with my champagne toast. Wow, that stuff really goes to your head when you don't have much in your system. The band started playing, and Jeff and I decided to ditch the Spam for the dance floor. Having had champagne and no food, we were less than coordinated. In fact, we were a mess. Jeff started telling me Spam jokes, and we both laughed uncontrollably and eventually fell into a room divider that was also a raised bed for plants. The entire thing crashed to the floor, dirt and flowers flying everywhere.

We were horrified. We ran.

We snuck out the back and went to the nearest place to get food at midnight in Minneapolis: Subway.

"Next time, we should really plan ahead," I said to Jeff, as we reflected on the evening.

DAY 18 DOSE OF FUN

> *Plan ahead for your day. Don't get sunburned, striped,*
> *soiled, spammed and starved at Subway*

MORE MAGIC

The tips I mentioned yesterday (Day 17, O is for On the Go) require some planning ahead. I can't emphasize enough how much easier and fun it is to spend a little time prepping and pre-packing healthy foods than to go hungry or resort to less healthy options. We will be learning about my favorite planning-ahead tool, the slow cooker, on Day 22. The slow cooker allows you take a few minutes in the morning so that you can come home to a yummy smelling house and a home-cooked meal. Most people don't know that your slow cooker can also be used overnight to prepare amazing hot breakfasts that are sure to be a family hit. I'll go ahead and give you a slow cooker breakfast recipe here that will have your morning kitchen smelling like apple pie.

But first, I want to invite you to listen to an interview I had with Juliette Britton, Registered Dietitian and course instructor at www.MakeNutritionFun.com. Juliette offers advice on how to plan your shopping lists, set up your pantry and fridge, and organize your week for optimal health. Please visit www.kathrynguylay.com/Juliette to get the downloadable interview delivered right to your inbox.

Recipe

· ·

Overnight Apple Pie Porridge

This recipe follows the Recipe Framework for Slow Cookers.

Ingredients:

Whole grains
- 1 cup uncooked steel cut oats

Fruits/veggies
- 2 apples, washed and chopped

Liquid
- 1 ¾ cups milk (or almond milk, rice milk or another substitute)
- 1 ½ cups water
- Seasonings
- 2 tablespoons brown sugar
- ½ teaspoon cinnamon
- ¼ teaspoon salt
- 1 ½ tablespoons butter (this is optional, but I like the flavor)

Toppings
  - ½ cup chopped walnuts, chopped almonds
  - Maple syrup, additional milk or butter, ground flax seed, if you like
  - Sliced bananas, raisins, dried cranberries or raisins

Directions:

Spray your slow cooker with olive oil spray. Combine everything above **except** toppings. You will add toppings once the dish is cooked in the morning. Cook in the slow cooker on low for about 7 hours, or if you make a double batch you can leave it at least another hour. If you are cooking this recipe overnight and you want to sleep longer (like me), just add more liquid (about ½ to 1 cup additional), and it will be fine for a nice, long sleep. Arianna Huffington would approve.

Day Nineteen

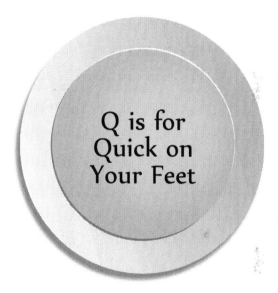

Q is for Quick on Your Feet

Question: What word might just stop you in your tracks in your quest for more home-cooked, healthy meals? It isn't even a bad word.

That word is *recipes*.

Recipes are great for learning how to cook or learning how to combine food elements. And, of course, recipes are essential to baking because making cakes, cookies, and pastries is more of a science.

Recipes, however, make you feel like you're locked into a certain set of steps. Don't have fennel seeds on hand? Don't have chipotle peppers in adobo sauce? Unless you don't mind running out to the grocery store at the last minute (which I very much dislike), your plans for a home-cooked meal might get thrown out the window.

The solution is to be quick on your feet in making substitutions and ingredient decisions based on your personal taste, your budget, and what you happen to have on hand. I'm asking you to take a more creative and artistic approach to your meals, where you have unlimited freedom.

Unlimited freedom can also lead to culinary disasters, so here is where the Recipe Framework comes in.

When Nurture created the Recipe Frameworks in 2008, we revolutionized the way cooking classes were taught. Recipe Frameworks give you a basic understanding of what elements you might like to combine (for example, a grain with a protein source, some vegetables, a healthy fat, and seasonings) to make a delicious, nutritious meal. Recipe Frameworks make healthy meal planning flexible, simple, and easy.

Here is an example of a Recipe Framework for breakfasts:

Breakfast Recipe Framework

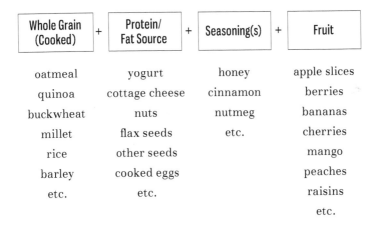

Whole Grain (Cooked)	+	Protein/ Fat Source	+	Seasoning(s)	+	Fruit
oatmeal		yogurt		honey		apple slices
quinoa		cottage cheese		cinnamon		berries
buckwheat		nuts		nutmeg		bananas
millet		flax seeds		etc.		cherries
rice		other seeds				mango
barley		cooked eggs				peaches
etc.		etc.				raisins
						etc.

We also created Recipe Frameworks for lunches and dinners, bean dips, soups, and breakfast smoothies. You can find all of the recipe frameworks at www.makenutritionfun.com/recipeframeworks.

These Recipe Frameworks were life changers for so many people, empowering them to start cooking and get back into the kitchen.

DAY 19 DOSE OF FUN

Make cooking fun with Recipe Frameworks;
you will benefit from the perks

MORE MAGIC

I encourage you to embrace cooking as an art. Embrace your inner artist when you are in the kitchen! Try on the artist persona in today's daily activities in the kitchen and see what you come up with. When I remind myself of my artist-side, pancakes get smiley faces, colors get arranged on the plate, and even cookie cutters come out to cut sandwiches or plate food in a most appealing way.

If you'd like some statistics about eating more veggies and how to make veggies cool, you can listen to a very short interview that I did with Lisa Davis on the Naturally Savvy radio show. Please visit www.kathrynguylay.com/naturallysavvy to get the downloadable interview delivered right to your inbox.

Day Twenty

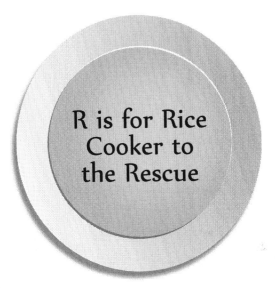

R is for Rice Cooker to the Rescue

Rice cooker: This little powerhouse of a cooking appliance is the victim of the worst product-naming snafu in the history of devices. Why? Because most people who happen to own a rice cooker think to use it only when they are making rice.

Big mistake!

My rice cooker sits on the counter as a most honored guest in my kitchen. In the spirit of its Japanese heritage, I've renamed my rice cooker *cooker-san*, or most honored cook. Many college students can tell you how to make everything from sautéed salmon (which I've done and enjoyed) to BBQ ribs (which I have not tried) in a rice cooker; however, it is whole grains, lentils, and split peas that follow the exact same rules as rice. There's no guessing and no slaving over the stove, watching pots that boil (or don't, according to the old adage). The cooker-san does everything for you, independent of your watchful eye!

Here are the simple steps to becoming friends with your own cooker-san:

- Step 1: Rinse the grains/lentils/split peas to remove dust and other particles. Grains can also be soaked overnight, making them easier to digest. If you decide to soak them, you can add a little lemon juice, because the acid helps break them down even more.

- Step 2: Measure using the 2:1 rule. For every cup of grains, lentils, or split peas, put in two cups of water.

- Step 3: Press down the on button. It will shift to the warm position automatically when the grains, lentils, or split peas are done.

- Step 4: Unplug it once the rice cooker clicks to warm. If you are a lazy cook like me, you can also leave the pot sitting there for a while on warm. Then, you are ready to make something yummy. Note that, when cooked, grains, lentils and split peas expand to two to three times their dry size.

- Step 5: Dress up those cooker-san goodies. Follow the Recipe Framework and add yummy spices and goodies that appeal to your senses.

DAY 20 DOSE OF FUN

Don't slave over the stove or pan; simply get out your cooker-san

MORE MAGIC

You are in for a surprise if you are looking for lots of ideas and inspiration to use your cooker-san. At Make Nutrition Fun, we have categorized our recipes by season, meal, cooking method, and allergy. Guess what! We have an entire category (under cooking method) dedicated to rice cooker recipes. We used the common street name (rice cooker) because that is what the world calls that piece of cooking equipment, whether we like it or not. Check out the recipes today at www.makenutritionfun.com and click on the box on the home page that says Recipes. You'll be taken to our amazing archives, where you can see just the type of recipes you are seeking. Enjoy!

Recipe

Sweet Potato Barley Salad

Ingredients:

- 1 cup of barley, cooked in rice cooker
- 1 medium sized sweet potato
- 1 can (15 ounces) black beans, rinsed
- ½ red bell pepper, washed and chopped
- ½ red onion, peeled and diced

For dressing:

- 2 limes, juiced (about ¼ cup)
- 3 tablespoons extra virgin olive oil
- 1 teaspoon chili powder
- ½ teaspoon ground cumin
- ¼ cup chopped cilantro
- 1 teaspoon honey
- ¼ teaspoon each salt and pepper

Directions:

Cook barley in the rice cooker. Allow pot to cool and rinse out for second use. Place barley in bowl and keep at room temperature. Peel and cut sweet potato into one-inch chunks. Place sweet potatoes on steaming rack in rice cooker. Add ½-cup water. Turn the rice cooker on and steam potatoes until button pops, about 10 minutes. While potatoes are steaming, make the dressing (combine all ingredients for dressing and whisk). Add sweet potatoes to the bowl with the barley and add all the remaining ingredients. Pour dressing over and gently toss. Taste for any additional seasonings. Serve warm or at room temperature.

Day Twenty-One

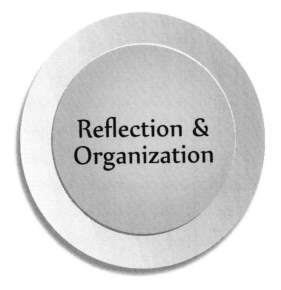

Reflection & Organization

Day Twenty-Two

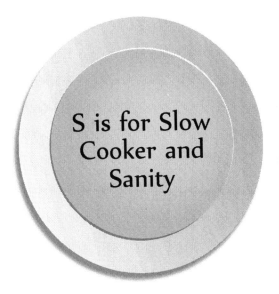

S is for Slow Cooker and Sanity

So, I might have solved some of your make nutrition fun challenges by introducing you to the cooker-san. But I know there are days when even the cooker-san is not the ultimate answer to the dinner dilemma because it still requires effort at the end of a long and tiring day.

Daily exhaustion and dreading the preparation of dinner are exactly what send many people to the local fast food joint or down the frozen dinner route instead of making a home-cooked meal.

My next solution for your health and sanity is the awesome and amazing slow cooker. This clever device allows you the flexibility to spend less than 15 minutes in the morning so that, when you get home at the end of the day, the house will smell of something delicious and inviting. The anticipation of something more nutritious and less expensive provides the willpower that perhaps you need in order to pass up fast food restaurants on the way home from work.

And, oh yes, the Recipe Framework is here for you again. So you can create slow cooker meals based on your personal preferences and what you can find in your kitchen.

Slow Cooker Recipe Framework

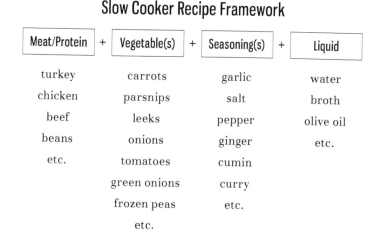

Meat/Protein	+	Vegetable(s)	+	Seasoning(s)	+	Liquid
turkey		carrots		garlic		water
chicken		parsnips		salt		broth
beef		leeks		pepper		olive oil
beans		onions		ginger		etc.
etc.		tomatoes		cumin		
		green onions		curry		
		frozen peas		etc.		
		etc.				

Here are some general guidelines for getting to know your slow cooker:

- Step 1: Add ingredients according to the Recipe Framework. Always be sure there is enough liquid in the recipe so as not to burn the meal in the slow cooker.
- Step 2: Plug in the slow cooker to a safe outlet. Cover and turn on the slow cooker. Guidelines are: Low setting for 8-10 hours (or overnight) or high setting for 4-6 hours. For animal proteins, use a meat thermometer to be sure it's done.
- Step 3: Turn to *keep warm* if waiting to serve.

You always can make larger quantities to freeze for the future or use leftovers for lunches or the next day's meals.

DAY 22 DOSE OF FUN

A slow cooker is your best friend,
for a home-cooked meal at day's end

MORE MAGIC

You guessed it. At Make Nutrition Fun, we have an entire category (under cooking method) dedicated to slow cooker recipes. Check out the recipes today at www.makenutritionfun.com and click on the box on the home page that says Recipes. You'll be taken to our amazing archives where you can find the recipes you are seeking. Enjoy!

Recipe

• •

Veggie Burrito Bowl

Ingredients:

- 1 cup frozen corn
- 1 can (15-ounce) black beans, rinsed
- 2 cups salsa
- 1 red or yellow bell pepper, seeded and diced
- 1 zucchini, sliced
- 1 summer squash, sliced
- 4-ounces cream cheese, cut into ½ inch cubes
- 4 cups brown rice, cooked (in rice cooker, of course)

Directions:

Place all the ingredients, except the brown rice, in a slow cooker and cook on low for 4-6 hours. Serve cooked veggies over brown rice and sprinkle with cheddar or Monterey jack cheese, if desired. Quinoa can be used instead of brown rice. For added nutritional value, serve over a bed of mixed greens with sliced avocado and shredded cheese.

Day Twenty-Three

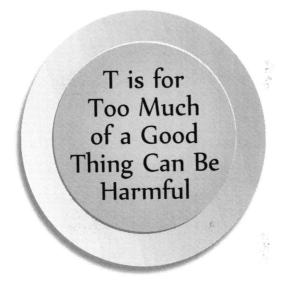

T is for
Too Much
of a Good
Thing Can Be
Harmful

The average teenager consumes an estimated 34 teaspoons of added sugar every single day. Sugar consumption is linked to such maladies as tooth decay, obesity, Type 2 diabetes, a suppressed immune system, and stunted growth due to too little vitamin and mineral intake.

The average American consumes 130 pounds of sugar per year, up from ten pounds in the 1800s and 40 pounds in the early 1980s. One third of all the carb calories consumed in this country come from added sweeteners. Of those, sugary beverages make up half.

I mentioned on Day Four (D is for Don't Be a Squirrel) that our bodies are hardwired to have a preference for sweet tastes. I also mentioned that, back when we lived in caves, this sweet tooth allowed us to seek out berries and fruits at the end of a long winter. Today, in a world with fast food and convenience stores at every corner, this inbred preference for sweets can backfire.

I encourage you and your family to cut back your sugar levels, starting with anything that is liquid and has added sugar in it. Then, start to cut down in other areas. Recognize that sugary foods cause a spike in your blood sugar and then a huge drop, leaving you feeling hungry and tired a few hours later.

Dr. Maria Maricich, Functional Medicine Doctor and Light Touch Chiropractor and a former U.S. Olympic downhill ski racer, believes that blood sugar fluctuations are one of the root causes of our society's health decline, including reduced brain function. Maricich likens rapid blood sugar fluctuations to taking your car and revving it up (high blood sugar) and then slamming on the brakes (low blood sugar). Over time, the result is a worn-out car or a worn-out body.

DAY 23 DOSE OF FUN

> *Sugar consumption is like a runaway train,*
> *damaging for you body and brain*

MORE MAGIC

Today, I'd love for you to visit a website that should be part of every school's health curriculum and something that every parent and child is aware of: www.sugarstacks.com. It demonstrates, through powerful visuals, how much sugar is in items such as beverages, candy, cookies, sauces, and many other items. The powerful methodology is based on the fact that each teaspoon (and each sugar cube) consists of four grams of sugar. The website shows pictures with the food item next to the number of sugar cubes (often stacked up in ominous pyramids) it contains. On Nutrition Facts labels, sugar is shown as grams, which most people can't immediately visualize. But when you take a candy bar that has 28 grams of sugar and place seven cubes (28 divided by four equals seven) of sugar next to it, the amount of sugar in foods starts to become very clear. Visit the website and see what surprises you!

Day Twenty-Four

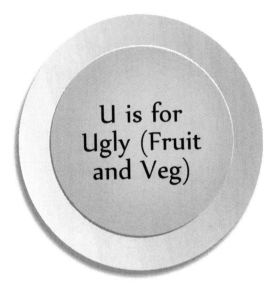

U is for Ugly (Fruit and Veg)

I learned about the brilliant Ugly Fruit and Veg campaign when I was interviewed by Marjorie Alexander on A Sustainable Mind podcast in 2016. Jordan Figueiredo, who started the Ugly Fruit and Veg campaign on the side of his waste management job in California, was a guest on the show just a few episodes before me. The Ugly Fruit and Veg campaign taps into an odd but true instinct that we have as humans to love and protect things that are so ugly that they are considered cute. The campaign utilizes funny, beautiful, and amazing images of less-than-perfect produce to highlight the fact that up to 40% of all produce goes to waste because of strict grocer aesthetic standards. Ugly Fruit and Veg posts on Facebook, Twitter, and Instagram and has a monthly reach in the millions. When I need a pick me up (or want to make my kids giggle enough that maybe they'll feel sorry for the sad-faced Kohlrabi that they'll actually try it), I go on to Ugly Fruit and Veg for inspiration.

DAY 24 DOSE OF FUN

*Odd shaped and otherwise waste,
these fruit and veggies are fun to taste*

MORE MAGIC

Try out if ugly works for you. I have seen the ugly factor break down the pickiest of eaters. Food struggles and picky eating usually are rooted in power struggles and the resulting negativity around food. Ugly Fruit and Veg photos bring out laughter and positivity to dissolve the negativity and barriers. Give it a shot. Maybe the peaches that look like butts won't solve your problem, but you might have luck with heart shaped purple potatoes and monster-like squash. See what makes a family laugh hard enough that you just might eat it.

To listen to Jordan's interview on the A Sustainable Mind podcast, please visit www.asustainablemind.com/011-jordanfigueiredo/.

To listen to my interview on the A Sustainable Mind podcast, please visit www.asustainablemind.com/019-kathrynkempguylay/.

Recipe

. . . .

Banana Soft Serve

Bananas get brown and ugly, and that's the best time to make Banana Soft Serve!

Ingredients:
- Ripe bananas, frozen
- Any other add-ins you can dream up (almond butter, frozen berries, nuts, etc.). See variations listed below.

Directions:

Slice ripe bananas into quarter-sized pieces and place them in an airtight bag in the freezer. Within a few hours, they will be frozen. Place the equivalent of about one banana (slightly defrosted) into a food processor. Process until smooth. The result: OMG, so good.

Variations to get you started:

Pineapple and Macadamia Nuts. Top with a few chunks of freshly sliced pineapple and chopped macadamia nuts.

Strawberry Chocolate. Add 1 cup frozen chopped strawberries to the food processor. Once processed, stir in ½ cup dark chocolate chips (or carob chips, or cacao nibs).

Cherries and Dark Chocolate. Top with a couple spoonfuls of cherries and a sprinkling of chocolate chips or cacao nibs.

Cinnamon Sunbutter. Add 2 tablespoons sunflower seed butter and 1 teaspoon ground cinnamon to the food processor.

Mango Peach. Add ½ cup frozen chopped mango and ½ cup frozen chopped peach to the food processor.

Raspberry Almond. Add 1 cup frozen raspberries to the food processor. Once processed, stir in ½ cup chopped almonds.

Dark Chocolate Banana. Add 2 tablespoons of dark chocolate sauce to the food processor.

Apple Pie. Simmer chopped apples with cinnamon, cloves and nutmeg (or cook them in the rice cooker!). Let the apple sauce thicken and cool, then pour over banana soft serve.

Strawberry Pistachio. Add 1 cup frozen chopped strawberries to the food processor. Once processed, stir in ½ cup chopped roasted, unsalted pistachios.

Blueberry Banana. Add 1 cup frozen blueberries to the food processor. Once processed, top with a sprinkling of chopped walnuts or almonds.

Day Twenty-Five

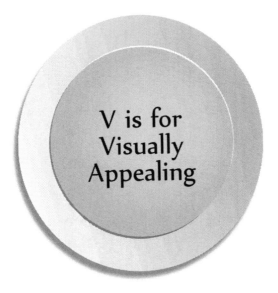

V is for Visually Appealing

Vegetables and other healthy foods can also be beautiful.

The art of plating is an important element of a chef's culinary education. "We eat with our eyes first," says David Wynne, Culinary Arts instructor at The Art Institute of Seattle, about food presentation and food plating. Don't worry, for home meals, a course in food plating is not required. But knowing how to approach edible art is.

How it works:

1. Choose a few foods. For picky-eater kids, make sure there is at least one food that you know your child will eat.

2. Depending on the age of your child, pre-cut the food or allow him or her to create their own shapes using a butter knife or cookie cutter.

3. Provide some support materials such as toothpicks, straws or skewers. Some designs will need 'glue': I find that nut butters and hummus are excellent adhesives.

4. Participate in the fun and encourage snacking as you and your young artist design an edible masterpiece.

5. Name your artwork. In a study, kids eat twice the amount of "x-ray vision carrots" as regular carrots. Other fun names include "super-hero spinach" and "magical trees" (for broccoli).

6. Place your masterpiece toward the right hand side of the plate. Items on the right are perceived by the brain as more appealing. Weird, huh?

DAY 25 DOSE OF FUN

Goofy food faces and edible mates,
are likely to vanish on picky kids' plates

MORE MAGIC

Research indicates that children need to be exposed to a new food fifteen to twenty times before they're willing to try it. Start getting your kids used to food using visual cues, which include books with real photography, as well as tactile exposure. Yes, that means getting kids to touch food; and one of the best ways to do so is to start a family garden. We'll go into more detail about family gardening on Day 29.

If you'd like to listen to a fun interview I did with Kathy Hart of WTXM on her Healthy with Hart podcast, we discuss naming foods to make them more appealing, what to do if your child doesn't like a particular vegetable or fruit, eating healthy on a budget, and beginner tips for gardening. Please visit www.kathryn-guylay.com/HealthyWithHart to get the downloadable interview delivered right to your inbox.

Day Twenty-Six

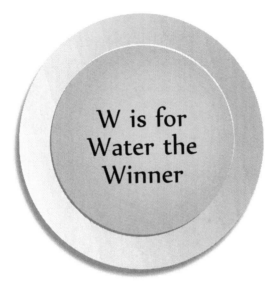

W is for
Water the
Winner

Why do we need to hydrate? Dehydration causes headaches, hunger, upset stomach, crabbiness, fatigue, and difficulty concentrating. Our bodies are comprised of more than 60 percent water. Proper hydration regulates body temperature, transports nutrients to our cells, and protects organs and tissues. Water also removes waste. Staying hydrated is one of the most important things we can do for our health.

What are our options for staying hydrated? With kids, I like to have them compare beverage choices and to give each one a prize. Just like the Olympics, we have bronze, silver, and gold medals.

First, we look at soda. We see that soda provides no nutritional value. It is loaded with sugar and sometimes caffeine. It is estimated that the average American consumes 592 cans of soda per year—and the 32-plus pounds of sugar that go with it! While diet sodas don't contain sugar, they also provide no nutritional value and contain many artificial ingredients that can be harmful to bodies and brains. It is best to limit soda to a *sometimes* or, better yet, *never* beverage. Soda doesn't get any medal at all.

Sports and energy drinks don't make it to the podium either. Many people think that sports drinks are healthy, but they contain a lot of sugar, artificial ingredients, and dyes. The electrolytes found in sports drinks are only needed when people are being so active that they sweat for an hour or more. If your kids need to replace electrolytes, then I recommend drinking water and taking an electrolyte replacement tablet. That way, they can stay hydrated and replenish their electrolytes without the artificial ingredients, sugars, and dyes found in sports drinks. You can also offer your kids water with a squeeze of fruit or veggie juice and maybe a pinch of salt, if they've really had a sweat fest. All fruits and veggies provide potassium, a key electrolyte; bananas are standouts when it comes to this mineral, and coconut water is an even better source.

When we get to fruit juice, we are now on the podium, but juice only comes in as the bronze medal winner of what we call the *better beverages*. Real, 100 percent juice contains vitamins and minerals but also a lot of natural sugar, so limit to no more than one six- to eight-ounce cup per day. Keep an eye out for juice look-alikes that are not 100 percent juice. Look past the marketing and read the ingredient list to make sure the drink is not a fruit or veggie wannabe.

Milk (but not chocolate milk) is our silver-medal winner for better beverages. Milk contains calcium and vitamin D, which help build strong bones and teeth. Not everyone tolerates milk well, so kids should listen to their bodies and tummies to make sure that milk agrees with them.

The gold medal goes to water! Water gives you a long-lasting hydration boost and contains no sugar, dyes, or artificial ingredients. The best part about water is that it is usually available and free.

DAY 26 DOSE OF FUN

When thirsty, reach for H20, the gold medal way to go

MORE MAGIC

If kids understand that water is the number-one choice but still want something special to dazzle the taste buds, I recommend *wuice*: water with a little bit of juice added from any fruit or veggie. For a flavorful refresher, add cucumber rounds, citrus slices, watermelon cubes, or berries.

Day Twenty-Seven

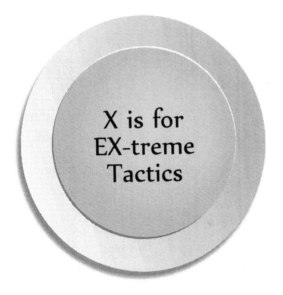

X is for
EX-treme
Tactics

X-Men with baby carrot machine guns?

Extreme tactics must be counteracted with extreme tactics. Advertisers prey on our children to get them to eat fast foods and processed foods. During the Super Bowl, companies pay $2 million to $3 million for every 30-second ad. The junk food and sugary beverage industries spend over a billion dollars a year on advertising.

Children are exposed to over 20,000 advertisements per year, about 55 ads per day. Jingles and phrases from ads seem to embed themselves in our memories. Companies utilize many tactics such as catchy jingles, endorsements by famous athletes or musicians, or free toys to attract young consumers.

Advertisements can't lie, but they don't have to disclose the whole truth. For example, a fruit punch beverage may have an advertisement or wrapper with images of fresh fruit. However, if you look at the ingredient list it may not contain any or may contain just a very small amount of real fruit juice. In order to know exactly what you're getting, it is important to read the small print, such as nutrition labels or ingredient lists. Teach your kids to be on the lookout for those sneaky little phrases like "PART of a healthy breakfast," and soon your kids will be making fun of, not being swayed by, sugar cereal ads.

You can also expose your kids to ads for healthy foods that don't have the budget to air on TV but can get their ads on YouTube. If you search "Baby Carrot Ad" on YouTube, you'll find a 30-second video created by a bunch of carrot farmers, namely Bolthouse Farms and nearly 50 other carrot growers, as a counter-attack on the snack foods industry. A $25 million campaign, this ad uses a lot of the same kinds of visual tactics that junk food companies utilize. The kids love the machine gun shooting baby carrots and the character that catches a baby carrot (bullet) in his teeth. I show this video to classrooms that I visit, and then I serve the kids baby carrots. They gobble them up.

DAY 27 DOSE OF FUN (which won't make sense until you watch the baby carrot ad)

A prehistoric bird and a carrot-shooting gun, extreme tactics make healthy food fun

MORE MAGIC

Soda is one of the most heavily advertised products in the world. To combat this giant, a grassroots campaign by kids and families was coordinated by the Center for Science in the Public Interest (CSPI) to "pour one out" – a campaign to replace sugary drinks with water. This counter-attack on the sugary beverage industry held a video contest to spread the message about the health dangers of sugary drinks. The winner was a rap by a family in Nashville, TN, inspired by the dad's personal struggle with soda consumption. You can find this video by searching on YouTube "Just pour it out video contest entry". You might find the music catchy and find yourself humming the tune as you guzzle water throughout your day.

Day Twenty-Eight

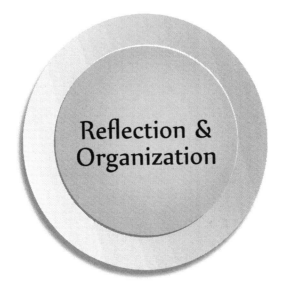

Reflection &
Organization

Day Twenty-Nine

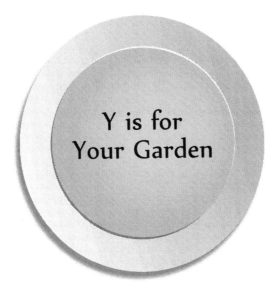

Y is for
Your Garden

Years before I started Make Everything Fun and Make Nutrition Fun, I wrote a blog called the Healthy Kids Ideas Exchange. There, I hosted a small community of bloggers with expertise in nutrition, food, and gardening.

One of my favorite posts was the Vegetable Gardener's Story by Elizabeth Matlin, a master gardener. I want to share some of the highlights with you here. My hope is to inspire you to try growing some of your own food, even if that means a tiny little pot of rosemary on the windowsill. There is no better way to get kids to eat healthy foods than to involve them in growing it.

THE JOYS OF DIGGING IN THE DIRT

Have you ever plucked a ripe tomato from the vine? Or tugged a plump rosy radish from the Earth where you had planted a small seed? If so, you know the rewards of growing your own vegetables. Whenever I step into my vegetable garden, I feel happy—the kind of happiness children experience in simple, everyday things. It is my playground, where I am in the present moment. Past and future disappear, and I am both energized and at peace.

So that gardening can become a joy for your entire family, here are a few pointers for first-time gardeners:

Start small: There's a fair amount of time and muscle that goes into planting, maintaining, and harvesting a garden. As with most lifestyle changes, it's essential to start small and gradually incorporate gardening as a new activity into your schedule. If your garden is too large to easily maintain, it may become a disappointing burden rather than a positive adventure. Expand your garden space gradually each year.

Make a plan: Keeping a simple record of what you plant from year to year is a useful tool as your garden evolves. In a journal or on a computer, draw a basic outline of your garden space and fill in areas with the names of the vegetables you plant. You might also include:

- Specific varieties, such as atomic red carrots or springer spinach
- The planting and harvesting dates
- Notes and comments on likes and dislikes, results, etc.

Share the experience: Ask the whole family to participate. Let your children select some of the seeds and plants. Young children can help plant seeds, pull weeds, water, and harvest small items, like cherry tomatoes and strawberries. Older children can each be assigned a small section to plant and maintain, even cooking their harvest for all to enjoy.

DAY 29 DOSE OF FUN

To be a healthy eating guide, grow a garden in or outside

MORE MAGIC

If you aren't convinced about the power of gardening, here are some additional proven benefits:

- **Physical activity.** I call it garden yoga. You work muscles in ways only gardening can provide. Balance, strength, and flexibility are enhanced.

- **Mental Health.** Connecting to nature and the Earth is a basic human need that most of us are not exposed to often enough. Gardening provides more than fresh air and sunshine. It reminds us how we are linked to nature and provides stress-busting therapy. It is a form of meditation.
- **Community.** Many neighborhoods have community gardens, where you can rent a plot of land for a very small amount of money. These plots not only provide ideal soil and sun, but you and your kids benefit from interacting with other passionate gardeners and their kids.

If you'd like to hear some inspiring stories about how gardening can help children physically and mentally, I suggest listening to an interview I did with child psychologist and expert in therapeutic gardening, Dr. Charles Majuri. One of the stories he tells in our interview is about a child who hadn't spoken in years, due to emotional trauma, and how the garden brought her out of her protective shell. Please visit www.kathrynguylay.com/GardenTherapy to get the downloadable interview delivered right to your inbox.

Day Thirty

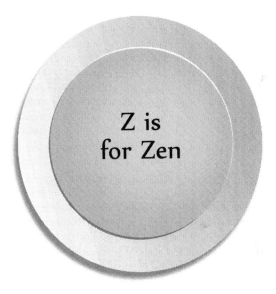

Z is
for Zen

Zen. You're at the end.

You've made it through a month of advice on how to make nutrition fun, and perhaps your mind is swirling with things to do and accomplish. I really hope you're not stressing out about buying supplies or, thanks to the advice in yesterday's Y is for Your Garden, out in the burning sun cutting through dry soil to try to get an orchard planted for harvest time. Remember, this book is about FUN. One of the best recipes for fun—or frameworks, since I don't always rely on recipes, as you know—is something I learned from my mentor, Marci Shimoff. It's called Intention, Attention, No Tension.

Intention means setting a goal or determining a direction that you want to go. For example, an intention for you as you read this book might be to improve the eating habits of your entire family.

I love the story of Jim Carrey, a well-known believer in the law of attraction, who wrote a check for 10 million dollars to himself at the age of 28 when he was still struggling as a young comedian. In the memo, he wrote, "For acting services rendered." He kept it in his wallet until he cashed it five years later, when he earned 10 million dollars for his role in *Dumb and Dumber*.

But Jim has been quoted as saying, "You can't just visualize it and then go eat a sandwich." That is the process of attention. Yes, you have to work at moving towards your intention. For someone reading this book with the intention of improving family eating habits, attention would be trying the tips in this book, applying the More Magic sections (and listening to the downloadable MP3s), and experimenting with the Recipe Frameworks.

Then it's time for no tension. Marci Shimoff reminds us that this part of the formula is where the magic really happens. When we push, push, push, we tend to create our own self-imposed roadblocks. If you push your agenda of healthy eating on your family and beat yourself up when you don't follow guidelines for yourself, you are creating tension. You need to apply a little Zen to the process of making nutrition fun.

Here are some actionable tips for bringing more Zen into your Make Nutrition Fun journey.

Plan meals and shopping in a neutral, private place. The grocery store, with its tactics to entice with cartoon characters, colorful packaging, and strategic placement, is not the place to negotiate what's for dinner tonight. Avoid power struggles around food by involving children and giving them choices by shopping and planning meals in a neutral and relaxing place like the kitchen table, when no one is overly hungry and, therefore, crabby.

Ask your kids, "What do YOU think we should we include on our shopping list this week?"

Use pictures of healthy foods, like food cards, and have kids sort out the things they'd like to buy. Maybe the fourth or fifth time looking at pistachios on a food card will be the time when your child decides to give them a try. Remain neutral yourself and ask your child to follow a simple rule about sorting through foods: "Please do not call anything 'yucky'; that is hurtful and not allowed."

Using neutral or interesting descriptions, such as "that kale looks bumpy" or "that watermelon looks juicy," is perfectly fine and should be encouraged.

Turn your "problem" child (or spouse) into the "solution." Like everyone else, kids (and spouses) love to feel valuable and needed. Take over the problem yourself and ask your child to help you!

"Mom really wants to eat more dark orange veggies because she heard that they are really good for her eyes and hair. Can you help Mom find some dark orange veggies that will be good for her?"

Or, "Dad learned that Olympic athletes eat lots of blue and purple fruits and veggies for energy, and he wants to be able to finish that race he signed up for. What would you suggest?"

When given a problem and some empowerment, you won't believe how your child will run to find butternut squash, blueberries, and eggplant and maybe just try them along with you!

DAY 30 DOSE OF FUN

When you really, really want to make it so,
sometimes the best thing to do is just let go

MORE MAGIC

Perhaps you'd like an inspiring story to demonstrate how the process of intention, attention, no tension really works. I suggest listening to Marci Shimoff's story of how she came up with the *Chicken Soup for the Women's Soul* series by applying the formula of intention, attention, no tension. Please visit www.kathrynguylay. com/Marci to get a downloadable interview delivered right to your inbox.

Listen while you're out for a walk or jog, while doing errands, or even cooking.

Have fun.

Acknowledgments

It is with great delight that I take this opportunity to express my gratitude for so many individuals and groups who have helped me on this journey. Writing a book is similar to the many other creative processes in my life, one based on collaboration and teamwork.

I want to especially thank my family: my incredibly supportive husband, Jeff, and my bright and energetic kids, Elena and Alexander. Thank you for letting me share with others some of our family stories about how we make nutrition fun. I also want to thank my dad, Robert, for being an incredible role model in the health field and for being an encyclopedia of knowledge. To my mom, I send a big hug of appreciation and love for the times we spent in the kitchen together carrying on the traditions of the Baranowski family.

Within these pages, I've shared with you the stories of my work at Nurture. This organization – and its volunteers, participants, and donors – has made a profound difference in my life and has contributed to the book's content and supporting resources. To learn more about Nurture, I invite readers to visit www.nurtureyourfamily.org and consider supporting our mission.

I also want to thank my extended family for being so amazing. Thank you for reminding me to "keep it fun," which is consistent with my brands: *Make Wellness Fun*, *Make Nutrition Fun*, *Make Publishing Fun* and all the other areas in which I intend to put a little more fun in the future under the parent organization *Make Everything Fun*.

August 2017

About the Author

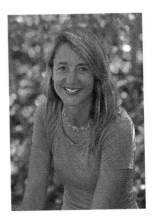

Kathryn Kemp Guylay is a speaker, certified nutritional counselor, coach and educator with a master's degree in business administration (MBA).

Kathryn was named a 2016 and 2017 "Woman of the Year" by the National Association of Professional Women.

The award-winning and bestselling author of five books, she is on a mission to help others be happier, healthier and more productive.

As a sought-after nutrition, wellness, publishing, and business expert, Kathryn is often interviewed by leading media, such as ABC, CBS, and NPR, and hosts two podcasts: *Mountain Mantras: Wellness and Life Lessons* and *Positive on Publishing*.

Kathryn's books to date include:

- *Mountain Mantras: Wellness and Life Lessons from the Slopes*
- *Give It a Go, Eat a Rainbow*
- *Where Does a Rainbow Grow?*
- *Look Before You Leap: The Smart Author's Guide to Avoiding the Money Pit and Achieving Financial SUCCESS in Publishing*

More information about Kathryn's products and services can be found on the following pages.

To continue to be in touch with Kathryn, please visit www.MakeEverythingFun.com for her blog posts and sign up for her free newsletter.

About *Make Nutrition Fun*

Continue the fun journey to make healthier eating part of your every day life through

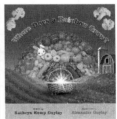

- delicious recipes
- nutrition resources, and
- online education.

Learn more at www.MakeNutritionFun.com

Entertain, Educate, and Engage Young Children with the *Eat a Rainbow* Series

"Teaching kids where our food comes from is an extremely important part of establishing healthy eating patterns at a young age. Sammy the bunny from *Where Does a Rainbow Grow* is the perfect ambassador to take young readers on a magical journey to learn how to identify plants as healthy food sources. Students are already connected to the main character, Blake, and love to be reminded how each color group from Mother Earth helps our bodies and gives us energy. An important addition to school and home libraries."

—Chef Ann Cooper, internationally recognized author, chef, educator, speaker, advocate for healthy food for all children and founder of the Chef Ann Foundation

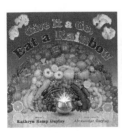 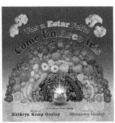 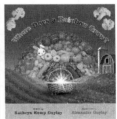

| Main theme: Eating fruits and veggies is fun and gives your body energy. | Spanish edition of *Give It a Go, Eat a Rainbow.* Coming soon: Spanish edition of *Where Does a Rainbow Grow?* | Main theme: A healthy rainbow of food comes from Mother Earth and plants. |

To learn more, visit: www.GiveItaGoEataRainbow.com

About *Make Wellness Fun*

Guiding you to peace and balance with expert advice through the "Mountain Mantras" podcast and online learning resources.

Learn more at www.MakeWellnessFun.com

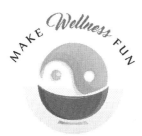

"Kathryn is a **national leader** for her work to create better health in our nation."

—Dr. David Holmes, Head of School Emeritus; executive director of Strategic Initiatives at Community School of Sun Valley, Idaho

"The wellness movement is gaining more and more strength today, thanks to **leaders like Kathryn**."

—Elisabeth Grabher, Board President of the Sun Valley Wellness Festival

"As a devoted advocate for lifestyle as medicine and an ardent, lifelong skier—this book beautifully conjoins two of my passions. There is expert guidance through the bumps here—with wisdom, experience, and humor on abundant display—and the turns, all well carved. Skiers and eaters will find this an empowering, illuminating read."

—Dr. David Katz, founder of the True Health Initiative

About *Make Publishing Fun*

Inspiring your publishing journey with coaching and consulting, the "Positive on Publishing" podcast, and online courses.

Whether you suffer from writer's block, don't know where to start, or simply want a community to help you with your journey, the Make Publishing Fun community is here to help you.

Yes, at MPF, our mission is to *Make Publishing Fun*. Learn more at www.MakePublishingFun.com

"Thanks again for having me on [the Make Publishing Fun Summit], Kathryn—you're a great interviewer, and it was a lot of fun!"

—John Tighe, Bestselling Author, Podcaster, Online Marketing Expert, Entrepreneur, Speaker and Coach

"In just a short period, Kathryn had me set up with a focused publicity plan, including technical/mechanical details as well as a strategy and plan of action. So helpful and important when one is trying to get the word out about helping others and spreading a healing mission."

—Dr. Don St. John, author of *Healing the Wounds of Childhood*

"Your energy is very up-lifting. Thanks for all the resources."

—Geoff Affleck, #1 Bestselling co-author of *Enlightened Bestseller*, *Breakthrough!* and *Ready, Set, Live*

A final, humble but important request ...

Thank You For Reading this Book!

I really appreciate your feedback, and I love hearing what you have to say.

Please leave me a helpful review on Amazon, letting me know what you think of this book.

Just go to <u>Amazon.com</u> and type in "Make Nutrition Fun". When you scroll down to the reviews section, there is a grey box ("Write a customer review") that you can click on to share your thoughts. Thank you!

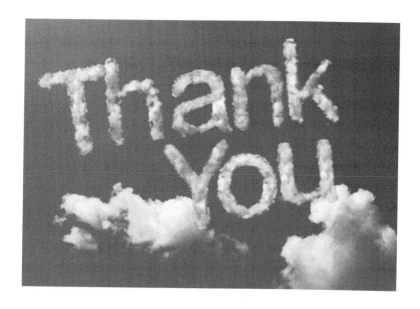